W9-ACV-628

THE COMING
CANCER
CURE

FRANCISCO CONTRERAS, M.D.

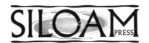

THE COMING CANCER CURE by Francisco Contreras, M.D.
Published by Siloam Press
A part of Strang Communications Company
600 Rinehart Road
Lake Mary, Florida 32746
www.siloampress.com

Unless otherwise noted, all Scripture quotations are from the New American Standard Bible. Copyright © 1960, 1962, 1963, 1968, 1971, 1972, 1973, 1975, 1977 by the Lockman Foundation. Used by permission. (www.Lockman.org)

Scripture quotations marked KJV are from the King James Version of the Bible.

Scripture quotations marked NKJV are from the New King James Version of the Bible. Copyright © 1979, 1980, 1982 by Thomas Nelson, Inc., publishers. Used by permission.

Scripture quotations marked NIV are from the Holy Bible, New International Version. Copyright © 1973, 1978, 1984, International Bible Society. Used by permission.

Cover design by Judith McKittrick

This book is not intended to provide medical advice or to take the place of medical advice and treatment from your personal physician. Readers are advised to consult their own doctors or other qualified health professionals regarding the treatment of their medical problems. Neither the publisher nor the author takes any responsibility for any possible consequences from any treatment, action or application of medicine, supplement, herb or preparation to any person reading or following the information in this book. If readers are taking prescription medications, they should consult with their physicians and not take themselves off of medicines to start supplementation without the proper supervision of a physician.

Portions of this book were previously published in *Health in the 21st Century* (Interpacific Press, 1997), 1-57946-000-3, and *The Hope of Living Cancer Free* (Siloam Press, 1999), 0-88419-655-0—both books by Francisco Contreras, M.D.

Library of Congress Catalog Card Number: 2002104352
International Standard Book Number: 0-88419-846-4

02 03 04 05 — 8 7 6 5 4 3 2 1
Printed in the United States of America

Dedicated to my father,

Ernesto Contreras, M.D.

A true "Quixote" who, for the love of his patients, bore all things, believed all things, hoped all things and endured all things.

The Preeminence of Love

by

Ernesto Contreras, M.D.

If I were to become a famous research scientist or renowned physician, and though I could display graduate degrees and prestigious diplomas; if I were considered an excellent teacher and dynamic speaker; but have not LOVE, I am nothing more than a sounding brass or a tinkling cymbal.

And though I were a gifted clinician, receiving great recognition for my diagnostic abilities, and if I could understand all the mysteries of the human body and have confidence that I can successfully treat any kind of disease—even cancer—but have not LOVE, I am a useless nobody.

And though I invest all my money to build the best facilities, buy the best equipment and employ the most prominent physicians for the sake of my patients; if I devote all my time to their care, even to the neglect of my own family and myself; but have not LOVE, it profits me nothing.

LOVE is an excellent medicine, prescribed with kindness; it is non-toxic; it does not depress the body defenses, but strengthens them.

LOVE mixes well with all kinds of remedies, acting as a wonderful positive catalyst to their healing powers.

LOVE relieves pain and maintains the quality of life at its highest level.

LOVE is easily assimilated by everyone; it never causes allergies or evokes intolerance.

Common medicines come and go. Those considered excellent yesterday are useless now. Those considered useful today will be worthless tomorrow. But as a medicine, LOVE has passed all the tests of time; it will be effective always.

Medicines we only understand partially, and most therapies are only experimental.

But the time will come when we understand absolute truth, and all doubt will cease in the face of LOVE.

Through LOVE our immaturity and stumbling efforts will vanish; we will establish great rapport between physician, patients and relatives, free from false motives and pride.

Today many truths appear as blurred images to us as physicians; we can't understand fully the spiritual influences in the practice of medicine; but the day will come when medical science will recognize how the Spirit works through LOVE to maintain life; then we will be true physicians.

And now there remain three powerful medicines for the spirit: Faith, Hope and Love; but the greatest of these is LOVE.

—ADAPTED FOR PHYSICIANS FROM
1 CORINTHIANS 13:1–13

≈

Dr. Contreras received his inspiration for this Physicians' Love Chapter in his Spanish language. It follows for those who can enjoy it as originally written.

La Preeminencia Del Amor

Por

Dr. Ernesto Contreras Rodríguez

Si llegara a ser investigador famoso o un clínico notable y obtuviera toda clase de diplomas y grados honoríficos; y si fuera conocido como un gran conferencista y maestro, pero no tuviera amor, vengo a ser como metal que resuena o címbalo que retiñe.

Y si tuviera el don de ser un clínico extraordinario, capaz de llegar a los diagnósticos más exactos; y si llegara a comprender todos los misterios del cuerpo humano; y si llegara a poder curar toda clase de padecimientos, incluyendo el cáncer, pero no tengo amor, nada soy.

Y si invirtiera todas mis riquezas en construir clínicas y hospitales suntuosos y los equipara con lo mejor que ofrece la ciencia médica; y si contratara los mejores especialistas para trabajar conmigo; y si ofreciera los cuidados más completos día y noche; y yo mismo me sacrificara dando muchas horas de mi tiempo a mis enfermos, pero lo hago sin amor, de nada me sirve.

El amor es una medicina incomparable y estimulante; no es tóxica, no es agresiva.

Se puede combinar con cualquier otro medicamento sin causar conflictos o efectos secundarios; es un maravilloso catalizador positivo.

Calma dolores y mejora la calidad de vida de los pacientes.

Es bien aceptado por todos; nunca produce intolerancias o alergias.

Medicamentos van, medicamentos vienen. Lo que se consideraba excelente ayer, ya no es útil ahora. Lo que es útil ahora será obsoleto mañana. Pero en la medicina el amor ha pasado las pruebas del tiempo y siempre será efectivo.

Porque la medicina sólo la conocemos en parte y la mayoría de los medicamentos son experimentales.

Mas llegará el tiempo en que conoceremos la verdad absoluta y nuestras dudas acabarán.

Por medio del amor nuestra inmadurez y nuestros titubeos se desvanecen. Gracias a él podemos entender y tratar a nuestros enfermos con toda propiedad, libres de sentimientos de falsa superioridad y orgullo.

Actualmente, las cosas del espíritu en la práctica de la medicina nos parecen inciertas y borrosas, mas pronto vendrán los días en que se reconozca por toda la clase médica la influencia del espíritu en el origen de las dolencias físicas y, entonces, seremos verdaderos médicos.

Ahora pues, consideremos que existen tres valiosos medicamentos del espíritu que tenemos a nuestra disposición: la fe, la esperanza y el amor. Pero el más eficiente de todos es el amor.

—Adaptado por medicos de
1 Corintios 13:1–13

Table of Contents

Section I—Cancer Is a Tumor?

Section III—Promoting Prevention

Section IV—Embracing the Cure

We Will Win Against Cancer!

The twentieth century will go down in history as the great epic of scientific breakthrough and technological advance. It is hard to believe that we began the 1900s without automobiles, electricity, telephones, computers, Internet and space travel.

Scientific "Miracles"

The medical field was profoundly impacted as well. We doctors once relied on patient-doctor relationship, intuition and folk remedies. But twentieth-century research gave us lasers, 3-D imaging, fiberoptic cameras (to go inside the human body and take a firsthand look) and an arsenal of pharmaceuticals designed to address just about every pathology. It is as if the physician's *messiah* arrived with such "miraculous" advances that we thought no pathology could escape our "divine medical wisdom."

The results? Acute medicine is at the top of its game. We are able to save lives and limbs like never before—great news for accident victims! Our trauma specialists and surgeons could even put Humpty Dumpty back together again.

Polio, smallpox and tuberculosis have nearly been eliminated in developed countries. And wow! It's amazing how advanced and even routine open-heart surgery has become. I think a lot of people have the mentality, "Why cut back on the pleasure of fried foods and smoking? If I have a problem, the doctors can fix it."

But then there is cancer...

No Magic Bullet?

We have always known in the medical community that the cure for cancer would be found through *research*. Scientists were so sure that they could find "the cure" for cancer if they were given proper funding. They made such a convincing case that they were able to gain federal support for their research. In 1971, President Nixon signed the National Cancer Act, which dedicated part of the national budget to cancer research through the National Cancer Institute. In spite of that national commitment to cancer research, the incidence and mortality rates of cancer have continued to increase each year since then.

Today, every twenty-four seconds of every day, someone in America is confronted with the diagnosis of cancer. In this new millennium, 50 percent of men and 30 percent of women in the United States are expected to develop some form of cancer at some time in their lives. Cancer is presently the second leading cause of death, exceeded only by heart disease. In the United States, cancer causes one out of every four deaths.[1] And these statistics are still on the rise.

Research money has been unable to buy the cure for cancer. "Why not?" you may ask. Part of the problem may be that we have been searching for the *cure* instead of searching for the *cause*. We have been treating the symptoms of the disease (tumors, for example) instead of treating the patient and his metabolic deficiencies that caused his body to succumb to disease.

Another obstacle may in fact be the scientific method of research. Science requires that each therapy be tested independently. If a therapy cannot demonstrate tumor destruction autonomously, it is discarded. In a sense, if a therapy is not a *magic bullet*, it is considered to have no scientific value. There is no consideration of the synergy that combined therapies might produce to fight the disease.

As a cancer surgeon, I know of no magic bullet. Conventional therapies such as chemotherapy, radiation and surgery often obtain objective results: the destruction of malignant cells. But they usually fail to address the other health needs of the patient to restore a quality

> **Research money has been unable to buy the cure for cancer.**

of life. That is why we see so many patients pass away even though there was initial response to the conventional treatment. In fact, most cancer patients die from the devastating side effects of the therapies, even when they effectively destroy or reduce tumor activity, and not from the malignancy.

Pioneering a Cure

My father, Ernesto Contreras, M.D., specialized in pediatric clinical pathology at the Children's Hospital in Boston.[2] As a founder of the Oncological Society and Pathological Society in Mexico, he was considered by the medical community to be one of the most promising doctors in his field. However, my father soon became discouraged with the poor results he was experiencing for healing his cancer patients using conventional methods of treatment.

I have been close to suffering patients since I was young. I was nine years old when my father—the best cancer doctor I know—decided to treat cancer patients with alternative therapies. Because of my childhood experiences with my father, at the age of fourteen I decided to become a surgeon.[3] Today, even the most orthodox practitioners of conventional medicine recognize the benefits these alternative therapies can bring to a patient. This was not true, however, when my father began to explore their healing potential. By 1963, he had been ostracized by the medical community because of his unconventional attempts to alleviate the suffering of cancer patients.

Although my father's progressive methods and healing philosophy have since gained wide acceptance throughout the medical establishment, at that time not one hospital wanted to provide the services he requested for his patients; not one colleague wanted to be associated with him. As with other medical pioneers before him, he was isolated and exiled from the medical community because he dared to challenge conventional methods of treatment for cancer.

None of this rejection by his peers impaired my father's passion for searching for alternative treatments for his patients who were victims of cancer. When his out-of-town patients needed hospitalization, which was refused them because they were his patients, he would bring them home. My sisters, brother and I were expected to relinquish our bedrooms for those hurting, dying people. In this way, our entire family was involved in helping patients to improve their lifestyle and to cope with the terrible realities of this disease. I saw their pain firsthand, and their suffering burdened me. I began to feel a deep desire to learn to heal them.

My Passion Birthed

These childhood experiences seeded the respect and appreciation I have for good health and nurtured within me a deep passion for healing those who are sick. At an early age I became painfully aware that life is very fragile and that there is no such thing as physical immortality. I knew I wanted to be a cancer surgeon like my father.

In my youth, I studied to make my dream a reality, first attending a Christian college in America and then a medical school in Mexico. When I was finally accepted as a cancer surgeon at the First University in Vienna, Austria, the finest medical school in the world, my childhood dream had become a reality.

The professors there were patient with me as I worked to

learn the German language on the job. They placed me in a position where language demands were minimal: in the operating room. As a result, I spent more time performing surgeries on cancer patients than did my German-speaking classmates. During one five-month period, I arrived at the hospital before sunup and left the operating room after sundown. These foundational years gave me excellent medical training in the con-

> **We must consider all options that can achieve tumor destruction without causing the patient's general health and quality of life to decline.**

ventional approach to medicine through my extensive surgical experience in oncology.

Founding Our Hospital

I believe the war against cancer in which we have invested our entire lives is one we will win; I've staked my life on it. I have been close to suffering patients since I was a boy in my father's home. I still consider my father the best cancer physician I have ever known. And I always knew that my destiny would involve treating cancer patients as my father so faithfully did. Ours is a generational destiny—filled with hope—that the tremendous progress my father advanced toward the coming cancer cure can be propelled forward in my lifetime.

My father's passionate quest and unbridled commitment for finding a cancer cure kept him pursuing alternative therapies, along with his use of conventional treatments, in his cancer-fighting strategy. Eventually, he founded the Oasis of Hope Hospital in Baja California, Mexico, where I am now the general director. I have worked with my father since 1983, and together we have become well known around the world for the successful treatment of cancer patients.

My father and I have shared the message that when it comes to cancer, we must consider all options that can achieve tumor destruction without causing the patient's general health and quality of life to decline. In adopting this metabolic therapy approach to treating cancer, we have positioned ourselves between the proverbial "rock and a hard place" in the medical community. Orthodox doctors have spoken out against us because of our use of natural therapies and vitamins. And alternative doctors have lashed out at us for our use of surgery, radiation and chemotherapy.

Our motivation has not been—nor is it now—popularity with peers; it is the well-being of our patients. So, we do not rule out any therapy option. If it will improve the patient's quality of life and his prognosis, we will use it. It is not what we use; it is *why, how* and *when* we use it.

For example, we rarely use chemotherapy. But in the case of metastatic cancer of the liver, we have found that by delivering 5FU chemotherapy directly to the tumor in the liver via a catheter that I surgically implant through the portal vein, we can significantly reduce the size of the tumors without all of the negative side effects associated with chemotherapy.

At the same time, we provide vitamin and nutrition therapy to preserve the patient's immune system, which has to do the healing work for a long-term recovery to occur. We also provide emotional and spiritual support to the patient, which has probably been the most differentiating aspect of our hospital.

Our ongoing research into the nature and characteristics of this disease is helping us develop specialized treatments for each patient, utilizing conventional and alternative methods to promote their return to health. We now oversee the treatment of more than six hundred cancer patients every year in the Oasis of Hope Hospital.

What I have witnessed all my life has convinced me that the cure for cancer is as complex as cancer itself. In spite of that complexity, if you are a cancer patient or otherwise impacted by this cruel disease, you can take great hope in the fact that you are living during an explosion of truly amazing and dramatic cancer breakthroughs.

We know more about cancer today than ever before. The medical community is experiencing a dramatic paradigm shift from the faulty thinking that treated cancer as a "tumor" to attacking it at its source as the systemic disease it is now known to be. And there is wider understanding of and acceptance for using a comprehensive approach to healing through combining conventional and alternative therapies for cancer patients on a case-by-case evaluation.

> We do not rule out any therapy option. It is not what therapy we use; it is *why, how* and *when* we use it.

Take the Challenge!

We at Oasis of Hope are still pioneering the effort to clear the air of past prejudice against certain cancer therapies and biased preference for other treatments. I truly believe that the cure for cancer is coming soon; in fact, it may already exist. I am dedicated to studying every therapy option available until we uncover what will help the vast majority of people to overcome cancer.

On June 5, the annual date for the Worldwide Cancer Day of Prayer, people around the world pray for the cure. The prayer that I lift up is that God would grant wisdom to researchers and doctors to find more effective treatments for cancer and to educate people more effectively in ways to prevent cancer.

Discovering an adequate way to manage cancer has to begin with being educated to all of the treatment options that are available and then being willing to use them in combination. It is vital that we accept the fact that "one size" does NOT fit all when it comes to cancer treatment. This book shares with you the most interesting aspects of cancer treatment and prevention that I have used successfully over the past few years. Many patients are already ridding themselves of cancer through these therapies.

To effectively promote the coming cancer cure, we must be willing to understand the nature of the disease, the successes and failures of medical science and the compromised motivation of "the money trail." We will have to be willing to make hard personal choices, take responsibility for our environment and open our hearts and minds to embrace faith and hope that will take us to the ultimate cure.

> I truly believe that the cure for cancer is coming soon; in fact, it may already exist.

If you are willing to take this challenge, I can promise that you will be inspired to genuine hope for your own life and for the lives of those you love in *The Coming Cancer Cure*.

—FRANCISCO CONTRERAS, M.D.

Section One

Cancer Is a Tumor?

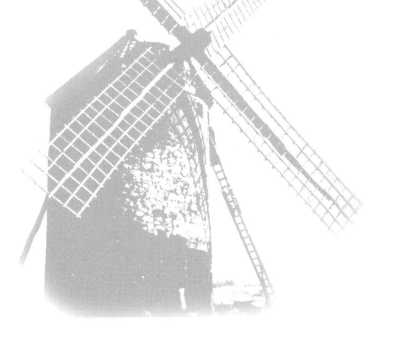

1 A Paradigm for Cancer Treatment

M y father, Ernesto Contreras, M.D., was one of the most promising residents to practice at Children's Hospital, which is a Harvard hospital, in Boston, Massachusetts. As a founder of the Oncological Society and Pathological Society in Mexico, my father was considered by the medical community to be one of the most promising doctors in his field. However, he soon became discouraged with the poor results he was experiencing for healing his cancer patients using the conventional methods of treatment—surgery, radiation and chemotherapy—in which he was trained.

After researching and implementing alternative treatments for cancer, which we later called metabolic therapy, my father was very encouraged with the improved results in his cancer patients. Then, in 1972 a World Congress on Cancer, convening in South America, invited him to present case studies of patients who benefited from his alternative metabolic therapy for cancer treatment. It is standard protocol in the medical community for the presentations made at these World Congress events to be published in the medical industry's most prestigious journals.

This was not to be the case with my father's presentation. A number of doctors raised objections to his presentation of alternative methods for curing cancer, stating they should not be included in a scientific journal. To address their complaints, my father was asked to present his case before a panel of oncologists at Sloan-Kettering Memorial Hospital who would determine if the science behind his treatment methods met the standards necessary to be published in a medical journal.

I accompanied my father to his presentation filled with excitement. I thought to myself, *It will take a miracle, but this might be the opportunity for my father's therapy approach to gain acceptance in the United States*. From the moment we entered the conference room, I knew what the outcome would be simply from observing the body language of the twelve doctors who made up this auspicious panel.

My father calmly began to present the first case study of the successful treatment of his cancer patient, displaying an x-ray that revealed the tumor size and location when he had first received the patient. When he displayed a later x-ray of the same tumor after the patient had undergone the treatment, one of the oncologists became so perturbed that he stood up and demanded that my father stop his presentation. This doctor then hurried out of the room and reappeared minutes later with a set of his own x-rays, which he began to display.

He challenged my father, "Look at this x-ray. Here my patient has tumors. We treated him. And as this next x-ray shows, the tumor is completely gone! In your second x-ray of your patient, it is clear that his tumor has actually grown!"

My father then asked the doctor, "How is your patient doing?"

The doctor replied, "He is dead."

Then my father said quietly, "Sir, you are quite right about my patient's tumor being somewhat larger after treatment. What you do not know is that this second x-ray was taken eight years after the first x-ray. And my patient was still living, working and enjoying life."

The oncologist retorted, "Your treatment methods cannot be considered successful because the patient's tumor was not eradicated."

It did not occur to this doctor that the results of my father's treatment, which lengthened and improved the quality of life of the patient, were more desirable than his own, which resulted in his patient's death. Incredibly, this oncologist who spurned my father's success inferred that the treatment of his own patient was successful because it eradicated a tumor, despite that fact that his patient had died.

For decades, the paradigm for cancer treatment based on successfully eradicating a tumor has resisted volumes of scientific research and case studies that prove the eradication of tumors merely treats a symptom of cancer, not the disease itself. And some conventional treatments that serve to eradicate tumors are so harsh and invasive they have become the cause of the patient's death rather than cancer.

This highly qualified specialist, who voiced the sentiment of the panel not to publish my father's presentation, was merely expressing the popular perspective of most specialists in the field of cancer. For them, success is not measured by the ultimate well-being of the patient; it is measured by the effective eradication of a tumor.

From where did this paradigm for treating cancer arise? As cancer raised its ugly head as a major disease early in the twentieth century, doctors treating the disease formed the foundation of thought defining the disease and its treatment for the medical community for decades to follow. Underlying its bias are historical perceptions of the disease as well as available treatments and, unfortunately, selfish motivations within the scientific community. The brilliant cancer specialists on that panel who censored my father were genuinely incapable of seeing the larger picture of successful treatments in terms of the health and well-being of the patient involved.

Historically, the medical community has considered cancer simplistically as a *tumor*. Unwittingly, we made the cancer tumor the object of our total focus, even to the exclusion of the well-being of the patient. The *classical* definition of a successful cancer treatment is *to destroy a tumor*. As a result of this paradigm for treating cancer, the overall well-being of the patient was of secondary concern.

Earliest Cancers: The Smoking Trail

Cancers caused by tobacco were some of the earliest environmental cancers to be discovered. It is here that we find the fertile soil from which we have harvested today's cancer epidemic. As far back as 1761, Dr. John Hill, a physician from London, began warning his patients that "an immoderate use of snuff" could cause cancer of the nose.[1] A few years later in 1795, German physician Samuel T. von Soemmerring noticed that pipe smokers appeared to be excessively prone to cancers of the lip.[2] Still, during the eighteenth century, cancer cases were extremely rare.

By the nineteenth century, more doctors were making the connection between cancer and tobacco. In 1858, Etienne-Frederic Bouisson, a French surgeon, recorded that of his sixty-eight patients with cancer of the mouth, sixty-three were pipe smokers.[3]

Early in the twentieth century, with the wholesale introduction of cigarette smoking for men and women, incidences of lung cancer began to appear on the scene. Until that happened, lung cancer was extremely rare.[4] Until 1898, only one hundred forty cases had been reported in the world medical literature.[5] As late as 1919 cases of lung cancer were still so rare that physicians were called in to observe a case of lung cancer, expecting it could be the only one they would ever see.[6] That expectation was short-lived.

In the twentieth century, tobacco caused the deaths of about 100 million people.[7] The World Health Organization has calculated that the 5.6 trillion cigarettes smoked per year at the close of the twentieth century will cause nearly 10 million fatalities per year by 2030. Today, lung cancer is the most common tobacco-related cause of cancer death.[8]

Roughly one-fourth of cancer deaths will be a result of lung cancer, and most will occur in developing nations as a result of cigarette companies' efforts to open new markets to offset declining consumption in industrialized nations.[9]

Although other cancers may have been on the scene far longer than the relatively recent advent of lung cancer, deaths by all cancers have only skyrocketed since the second half of the last century. The following shows the estimates of cancer victims in the United States alone for 2002:

> In 2002, there would be 1,284,900 individuals who would develop cancer and 555,500 individuals would die from it. The following are the types of cancer and its expected victims:
>
> - **Cancer of the digestive system**—250,600 individuals: 130,300 men; 120,300 women.
> - **Cancer of the respiratory system**—183,200 individuals: 100,700 men; 82,500 women.
> - **Cancer of the lung and bronchus**—160,000 individuals: 91,000 men and 69,000 women.
> - **Cancer of the breast**—205,000 women.
> - **Cancer of the prostate**—189,000 new cases: 30,200 men would die.[10]

The enormity of the impact of this disease is staggering, especially when we reflect upon its relatively recent arrival to the global health scene. And we need to understand that cancer treatment has evolved just as recently as the disease itself. Earliest treatments of cancer focused on the cancerous growth or tumor, as we have stated. Therefore, success was measured by the effectiveness of the treatment to eradicate that cancerous growth, whether or not the patient survived.

The Tumor and Its "Tentacles" Theory

Methods for cancer surgery that were established at the end of the nineteenth century involved mostly surgery for breast cancer. For these early surgeons, cancer was simply a deadly lump that needed to be removed. For them, the primary focus of the surgery was the speed with which it was performed because they had to operate without anesthesia or antibiotics.

Early in the twentieth century, surgical procedures improved with the scientific advances of ether, antiseptics, procedures and valuable instruments for checking the loss of blood. During this time William Halsted, considered to be the father of surgery in the United States, arrived on the scene. In Dr. Halsted's day, breast cancer was treated either by extricating the tumor itself or by removing the entire breast. Dr. Halsted visualized the disease as a tumor that grew by spreading cancer "tentacles" that reached into other parts of the victim's body.

Dr. Halsted was greatly influenced by Rudolph Virchow, a German pathologist, archeologist and anthropologist considered to be the pope of German medicine. Virchow had taught him that carcinogenic cells could not be spread through the blood stream. Cancer of the liver and lungs, they believed, arrived directly through these "tentacles" that reached various organs from a tumor.

This theory of how cancer was spread through the body (called "centrifugal dissemination") formed the basis for all future oncological surgery. These early cancer surgeons concluded that the maximum possible amounts of tissue in which such "tentacles" might be hidden had to be removed from the patient's body. Based on this faulty understanding, Halsted began to practice radical mastectomy, an operation that involved the removal of the entire breast and much of the surrounding tissue. His approach included the surgical removal of the entire infected breast, the adjacent muscles of the chest and all the lymph nodes in the armpit.

Halsted's radical mastectomy procedure gained wide acceptance in the United States and in Europe. His approach, together with his objectives and focus, became a teaching model for cancer surgery in the United States. Before long, this same philosophy and these surgical techniques were applied to other malignancies. The "tentacle" theory for the spread of cancer became the accepted paradigm of thought.

For example, surgeons of head and neck cancers developed what they called the "commando" operation. This severely mutilating surgery, named after a World War II technique for decapitating the enemy, resulted in the removal of the jawbone, the muscles of the neck and the blood vessels with their lymphatic ganglia. It could hardly be called a "cure."

The Tentacle Theory Challenged

The theory that cancer is spread through the body by "tentacles" was first questioned in 1910 by James Ewing of New York Memorial Hospital. He published evidence that contradicted the current paradigm of the "tentacle" theory. Dr. Ewing's evidence suggested that cancer cells could be spread via the blood stream.

His evidence showed that cancerous cells were spread to distant organs from the original tumor via the blood stream. Ewing's new theory (called "metastasis") constituted a cancer surgeon's nightmare. The eradication of a cancer tumor was still the sole focus of successful cancer treatment, but how could a surgeon be successful if it were true that cancer could freely travel through the bloodstream?

Despite this glaring new evidence that contradicted the need for removing massive areas of tissue surrounding tumors, the foundational paradigm of cancer surgery had been laid. Successful cancer surgery was still determined by eradicating a tumor and all its tentacles. Therefore, even after radical surgeries, when a cancer reappeared, surgeons continued to blame themselves for not removing enough tissue.

The tumor remained the focus of cancer surgery and was considered the source of cancer. As a result, surgeons continued developing even more radical surgical approaches.

A Cruel Controversy

During the next several decades, researchers compiled more evidence that contradicted the necessity of radical cancer surgeries.

In 1943, Frank Adair reported that sixty-three patients at Sloan Kettering Memorial Hospital who chose conservative surgery lived just as long as those who chose radical surgery. This evidence alone did little to alter the medical community's paradigm for cancer treatment reflected in Halsted's radical surgery.

Then, during the 1950s, a group of surgeons seriously questioned Halsted's radical surgery paradigm. George Crile of the Cleveland Clinic, a practitioner of radical surgery, was the first American physician to conduct a clinical trial for breast cancer using a conservative surgical approach. Most of his patients were given partial mastectomies instead of the deforming radical surgeries. He removed all of the cancer tumor and an ample margin of healthy tissue. Crile's results stood up to those obtained by radical surgery. But when he challenged the establishment with his data, he was censored as an extremist.[11]

In fact, cancer surgery became even more aggressive, and Halsted's mastectomy was amended and expanded. In addition to removing the entire breast, chest muscles and lymph nodes of the axillae, the "amended mastectomy" removed all the lymphatic ganglia under the sternum. This left the thorax of the patient looking like a washboard, because the ribs were now only covered by skin.

Leading cancer surgeons pressed for even more radical approaches. They introduced the "super-radical mastectomy" in which the patient's clavicle was fractured and the first rib removed, allowing doctors to cut out more tissue more easily. This procedure was soon abandoned after its results proved disastrous owing to the horrific psychological impact of the mutilation upon the patient.

The cruelty of cancer surgery would reach its zenith in the 1970s, when it occurred to Dr. Theodore Miller of the Sloan Kettering Cancer Center that the preferable method of fighting pelvic cancer was a hemiocorporectomy. This was a surgery that bordered on the macabre. Everything between the frontal and posterial rib cage—legs, pelvis and its organs, leaving only sufficient skin to form a pouch to contain the intestines—was removed, making it necessary to perform a colostomy (colon outlet connected to the skin) and nephrostomy (urine conduit connected to the skin) so that the patient could defecate and urinate through the skin.

It is believed that these patients died from emotional trauma, unable to accept themselves in their sub-human condition. This terrible procedure was the straw that broke the camel's back and predisposed us to practice more conservative procedures. Curiously, but tragically, it was surgical excess that set us on the road to moderation.

Questioning the Treatment Paradigm

In 1957, Bernard Fisher of the University of Pittsburgh organized a multi-institutional group called National Surgical Adjuvant Breast Project (NSABP). This group became key opponents of the general treatment consensus based on Halsted's paradigm of radical surgery. They submitted a series of studies successfully opposing Halsted's methods.[12]

Since Halsted strongly believed removing the lymph nodes was essential, a key NSABP study concentrated on case studies that involved the treatment of the lymph nodes. Surgeons treated more than a thousand women with mammary cancer. None of these women's cancer had spread to the lymph nodes in the armpit. The women were divided into three groups:

- Those treated by radical mastectomy
- Those treated by simple mastectomy with radiation therapy on the lymph nodes
- Those treated by simple mastectomy without radiation to the ganglia[13]

Approximately 18 percent of the patients treated experienced cancerous spread to the lymph nodes. The surprising thing was that the survival rate was the same for all three groups. *Radical mastectomy and radiation did not increase the survival rates*. The question to be answered was, why didn't it?

This clinical study went a long way to erode the credibility of the widely held understanding that cancer was contained to the site of the tumor and "tentacles" in the surrounding tissues. The spread of cancer began to be understood as cancer cells traveling in the bloodstream to other parts of the body and forming malignancies. This meant that eradicating a tumor was not the whole answer to the successful treatment of cancer.

The chart on page 11 shows how the treatment paradigm for cancer began to shift as a result of the NSABP's convincing case studies.

Members of Bernard Fisher's group (NSABP) were among the first researchers in the scientific community to view cancer as *a systemic disease that affects the health of the entire body* rather than as a tumor that could be cut out of a person's body. This was a dramatic shift in the popular paradigm for understanding the disease of cancer as a tumor. But it would still require many years for the medical community to begin to embrace this new paradigm for the treatment of cancer.

> ## Cancer is a systemic disease that affects the entire body.

Decades of New Ideas

The first sign of a shift in the treatment paradigm of the medical community was its focus on more gentle methods of treatment. During the decade of the 1960s there was increasing enthusiasm for conservative breast surgery. Many physicians leaned toward preservation of the breast, which meant that only the tumor was removed. This procedure was referred to as a local extrication, tumorectomy, lumpectomy or nodulectomy. When it was necessary to take away a part of the breast, it was called a partial mastectomy.

Halsted's Beliefs	NSABP's Findings
1. The bloodstream does not play a role in the spread of cancer cells.	1. The bloodstream acts as a highway for cancer cells to spread throughout the body.
2. Tumor cells are only spread by direct extension that occurs in an orderly manner.	2. Cancer cells do not follow an orderly pattern, but break away from the tumor and travel through the lymph nodes.
3. The network of lymph nodes acts as barriers to the passage of tumor cells and are not involved in the spread of the disease.	3. Lymphatic lymph nodes do not impede the passage of tumor cells; they often aid the spread of cancer. (Their infection is an indication of a weak immune system.)
4. Tumors grow and spread on their own; the patient's general health does not influence this process.	4. The general health of the patient directly influences every aspect of the tumor's progress.
5. Tumors will remain isolated and encapsulated inside the body for a long time.	5. Cancer is a systemic disease that affects the entire body, not just a particular location; cancer cells begin to circulate at a very early stage of the disease.
6. Specific surgical treatment is vital to patient's survival.	6. Local surgery has little effect on a patient's chances for survival.

In 1963, some physicians sought a balance between the two positions of radical and conservative breast surgery. They suggested the removal of the breast and the armpit lymph nodes without removing the pectoral muscles. This more aesthetically pleasing method, called a "modified" radical mastectomy, soon gained international acceptance.

In 1964, the first major scientific study supporting conservative surgery for breast cancer was initiated in Guy's Hospital in London. The study compared the removal of the tumor (local extrication) coupled with low doses of radiation therapy against radical mastectomy. It concluded that the life expectancy of patients treated with conservative surgery was the same as those who underwent radical mastectomies.[14] Criticism of this study was so fierce that the conservative movement suffered a costly setback.

During the next two decades, the 1970s and the 1980s, the doors were flung open to new ideas and novel ways of thinking regarding cancer treatment. The treatment of breast cancer especially continued to be a major topic of discussion in medical circles. Supporters of conservative therapies concluded that the recurrence of cancer in their patients was not eminent. Vera Peter of Toronto considered that, "although the rate of recurrence is significantly higher in patients treated with conservative surgery, their life expectancy is the same."[15]

In 1985, the NSABP published the first results of a comparative study of conservative surgical treatments (simple mastectomy, lumpectomy with post-operative radiation therapy) for breast cancer. The study concluded that patients treated with lumpectomy, the most conservative treatment of the three, lived as long as those who received one of the other two treatments.[16]

A Sad Commentary

George Crile, who we mentioned was the pioneer of conservative surgery in the United States, during the 1950s had dared to "look outside the box" of cancer treatment. During the

1970s, two decades before his death, Dr. Crile's theories about conservative cancer treatment had been amply confirmed to the medical community. Nevertheless, he never received any deserved recognition from the medical establishment for his progressive insights.

In his autobiography, the reader can hear a note of sadness in this regard. Dr. Crile wrote, "In retrospect it has been proved that most of what I said (concerning conservative cancer surgery) was correct. In spite of that, to my knowledge, not one of my critics has retracted a single one of their accusations."[17] Ironically, Dr. Crile died of lung cancer in 1992.

How is it possible that sixty years after the research proved that tumors do indeed spread by means of the bloodstream, we continue to drag our feet about changing our surgical criteria? There is very little difference between the oncology of the past and the current conventional cancer treatments. The focus for treatment is still primarily the tumor, and the main instrument for treatment is the scalpel.

While continuing to treat cancer with surgery to eradicate the tumor, oncologists developed radiation and chemotherapy as supplemental treatments. Once again, these treatments are aimed at the tumor with little consideration for the general systemic welfare of the patient. These treatments are a final attempt to blast away at any remaining cancer cells in the area of the tumor the patient may have. These treatment methods show that the paradigm of the medical community has not yet shifted to embrace fully the definition of cancer as a systemic disease; to these oncologists, cancer is still a tumor.

Chemotherapy

Oncologists realize that chemotherapy is the most toxic and least effective cancer treatment. In most cases, those patients receiving chemotherapy feel that they are dying. Many experience such severe nausea and vomiting that they must be hospitalized to help them endure the side effects of the treatment.

Other side effects they must suffer include their hair falling out and a loss of appetite.

The summary of the results of chemotherapy published in 1990 by Dr. Ulrich Abel, *Chemotherapy for Advanced Epithelial Cancer,* demolishes the credibility of one of the most solid pillars of orthodox oncology.[18] During his ten years as a statistician, Abel discovered that chemotherapy, the method used for treating the most commonly occurring epithelial cancers, which cause 80 percent of cancer deaths in the industrialized world, has rarely been successful. Epithelial cancers include cancer of the lungs, breast, prostate, colon and other organs.

Abel's summary affirms that there is no evidence that the vast majority of cancer treatments using cytotoxic drugs (chemotherapy) exert any kind of positive influence as far as life expectancy or quality of life are concerned.[19]

Listed below are Dr. Abel's results regarding cancers commonly treated with chemotherapy:[20]

- **Colon and rectal cancer:** There is no evidence at all that chemotherapy prolongs the life of patients suffering these malignancies.

- **Stomach cancer:** No evidence of effectiveness.

- **Pancreatic cancer:** The largest study was "completely negative." The patients who experienced prolonged life were those who did not receive chemotherapy.

- **Bladder cancer:** Chemotherapy is often applied but is not effective. No prospective study has been made.

- **Breast cancer:** There is no evidence that chemotherapy raises the chances for a patient's survival.

- **Ovarian cancer:** There is no direct evidence, but it might be worthwhile to research the use of platinum.

- **Uterine and cervical cancer:** There was no improvement in the survival rate of those treated with chemotherapy.

- **Cancer of the head and neck:** There was no benefit to receiving chemotherapy in terms of survival. There was the occasional benefit of reduction of tumor size.

It is true that sometimes these medications do, in effect, reduce tumor size.[21] But, according to studies, this tumor reduction has no significant impact in regard to improving the length or quality of life; sadly, in most cases, the side effects are the true source of a patient's nightmarish experience with cancer.

As a matter of fact, even when the tumor is reduced or eradicated, the cancer sometimes comes back more aggressively than ever. If 99 percent of a tumor is successfully eliminated, the resistant 1 percent remaining is often made up of the most aggressive cancer cells that will continue to spread the disease.[22]

A Legacy of Failure

The dismal failure of cancer therapies in the past is not the result of the procedures themselves. Rather, it is a result of the false premise on which treatment is based—that cancer is a tumor. Surgically removing tumors or destroying them through the use of chemotherapy and radiation without attempting to restore the organic deficiencies that caused the tumors to grow accounts for most cancer recurrences and deaths. Because cancer is a systemic disease, the overall health condition of the patient must be treated in order to assure long-term healing.

The second reason for past failure in cancer treatments is the result of a faulty definition of successful treatment. As we have explained, reducing the size or eradicating a tumor was the criteria for success, whether or not that resulted in a longer and better quality of life of the patient. When we accept the fact that cancer is much more than a tumor, that it involves a systemic breakdown in the patient's general health, then any of the treatments already discussed can be useful in aiding the healing process.

Diminishing a tumor mass or eliminating it completely, in some cases, can be helpful to aid the healing process when the cause of the disease is properly understood. However, the truth is that tumors are but a *symptom* of the metabolic failure of the body that allowed them to grow.

Treatment and Truth Triumph Together

An exciting dawn is breaking over cancer research and treatment as researchers unlock the fascinating secrets to what causes the metabolism to break down behind these metabolic failures. What is the true cause of cancer? How will that affect its treatment? As treatment and truth triumph together, they will resolve these essential, unanswered questions regarding cancer. Then we can expect to look back on the painful journey of this century in much the same way as our astronauts look back upon the past crude transportation of ox carts and clumsy farmer's wagons. The marvels of cancer treatment advances will cause us to rejoice together in the coming cure.

> An exciting dawn is breaking over cancer research and treatment.

2 A Paradigm Shift in Cancer Treatment

A century worth of research should bring forth some fruitful results, declared John W. Yarbro, M.D., Ph.D. from the National Cancer Institute. He continued, "Progress in cancer research in the 1980s has led to *predictions* of major improvements in cancer prevention and treatment in the 1990s."[1] His colleague Samuel Broder, M.D. reinforced the disappointment of the issue, stating that, "Although we are still searching for answers, the hallmark of the 1990s will be the application of research results from the '80s."[2]

These statements were delivered under duress because of the unfulfilled promise of the National Cancer Institute to find a cure for cancer by 1981. Instead, cancer incidence and the number of casualties continued to increase, as we have cited. Nevertheless, cancer research has given us vital information about cancer previously untapped. Advances in molecular biology, genetic engineering and other technological innovations have opened venues for treatment that had not previously been explored.

The failure to find a magic bullet to cure cancer brought a significant shift in the medical community's paradigm for the treatment of cancer. When the conventional methods of surgery, radiation and chemotherapy did not produce the desired results, some research scientists were willing to pursue other methods for treatment for cancer. It would require several books to explain all these exciting research developments. For our bene-fit, we will briefly discuss some of the most exciting research that has contributed significantly to the coming cancer cure.

Exploring a Tiny World

For those scientists who did not accept standard cancer treat-ments with their marginal "successes," the study of this enig-matic disease took them into a tiny world visible only at the molecular level. Willing to make a dramatic shift from the "can-cer is a tumor" paradigm, as my father had done years earlier, these researchers embraced the idea of cancer as a systemic or metabolic disease. That meant they had to look elsewhere for treatments instead of focusing on the scalpel and on radiation and chemotherapy.

And they would have to search for the true cause of cancer. Even in its very early stages they believed cancer had shown itself to be a systemic disease, not the localized condition (tumor) medical science once believed it to be. In other words, as cancer cells travel throughout the body via the bloodstream, they gain access to all the body's organs and tissues—even before serious symptoms of the disease are apparent. These brave scien-tists began to listen to an earlier pioneer who had dared to look at the "smaller" picture.

The voice of a prophet

Although some twentieth-century cancer researchers insisted on finding new ways to blast and chip away at cancer tumors, others were listening to a prophetic voice of long ago that had laid the foundation for cancer research of the twenty-first cen-tury and beyond. That prophetic voice was the work of Theodor Boveri (1862–1915) whose prodigious insights into the science of genetics and chromosomes form the foundation for today's startling cancer research discoveries.

In his chromosomal theory of heredity of 1902–1904, Boveri suggested that cancer tumors might be caused by tiny chromosomes that abnormally reproduce themselves, which is called the abnormal segregation of chromosomes to daughter cells.[3]

Boveri theorized that tumor growth is based upon a particular, incorrect chromosome combination that causes the abnormal growth characteristics of cancer cells. He suggested these characteristics are passed on during cell division from the parent to the daughter cells.[4]

Today's scientists understand that cancer cells are formed from normal cells that for some reason begin to grow out of control. Understanding the reason for this abnormal growth is the key to unlocking the mystery of cancer's causes and, scientists believe, a possible cure. Scientists want to learn what it is inside the cancer cells that make them grow out of control compared to normal cells that function correctly.

When they discover the "trigger" mechanism to this growth, scientists can then learn to shut down, block or disconnect these abnormal "triggers" or "messages" that energize the growth of cancer cells. This is the theory of present-day molecular cancer research in a nutshell.

Boveri wondered if the chromosomes held the secrets to these cancer cell growth-triggers. And although this information can only be viewed more deeply within the mystery of genes—at a microscopic level unheard of in his day, Boveri's instincts were absolutely right. He discovered what scientists are only beginning to understand today—that at a molecular level, cancer is nothing more than cells that for some reason begin to reproduce and grow abnormally.

Although Boveri died in 1915, his research convinced him that individual chromosomes carried different genetic information. In recent years scientists have been opening the door to genetic cancer research and walking through it—a door that was first discovered by Boveri, a prophet of today's cancer breakthroughs. The results of his research did not call for a shift from the "cancer is a tumor" paradigm; they demanded a completely new paradigm to define the disease.

Many of the concepts of today's genetic cancer research were foreshadowed with amazing accuracy in Boveri's writings, such as:

- Cell-cycle checkpoints
- Oncogenes
- Tumor-suppressor genes
- Tumor predisposition
- The relationship between genetic instability and cancer

Because of his prodigious insights, Boveri has proved to be a prophet whose voice proclaimed scientific truth so stunningly advanced for his time that scientists are just now beginning to understand its implications. The coming cancer cure is possible because of the cellular research advocated by Boveri that has yielded understanding of how a cancer cell is formed in a human body.

Discovering genes and DNA

Put on your lab coat, pull up a chair and adjust the focus of your high-powered microscope. You are about to take a look at the smallest level of life known to mankind: the amazing, tiny world that unlocks the secrets of genes and DNA. Our discovery will explain just how a normal, healthy cell becomes a monstrous, murderous cancer cell.

You may be aware that our bodies regenerate by cell division, the mechanism by which cells reproduce themselves. As we have stated, one parent cell divides in half, producing a new cell that looks and acts exactly like it. The new cell is often called a *daughter* cell. This cell division occurs millions of times in a person's body during his or her lifetime.

You may also be aware that inside the nucleus or center of your living cells are *genes* that contain a living blueprint for your life called *DNA*. Deoxyribonucleic acid, or DNA, is the universal alphabet for life. Amazingly, it only has four letters, and there is a lot of life around. Impossible?

If man will never exhaust music's possibilities with seven notes, imagine what God can do with a four-letter-word alphabet—certainly a lot more than dissonant sounds. The amount of information found in the DNA of just one gene could not be contained in all the books of all the libraries in the United States!

If you have blue eyes, it's because you received genes for blue eyes from your parents. You actually received a *pair* of genes, called *alleles*, for your eyes from your parents. Not all genes program the color of your eyes. Many different gene alleles exist that program your body for all its wonderful characteristics and functions. And one of these functions is to tell the cell when it is time to die. This tiniest level of all holds the secret of the mystery of life as well for how the disease of cancer develops its life.

A cellular mistake, and then…

Each time cell division occurs, there is a risk that a mistake can be made in the reproductive process of the new cell.

These mistakes can happen for different reasons: aging, harmful chemicals in the body, free radicals and a host of other variables. When cells fail to follow their precise genetically coded instructions for reproduction, they can become cancerous. While normal cells function and replace themselves though a fixed number of divisions during a natural, limited life cycle, and then die, cancer cells act very differently.

These cells become monsters that are actually immortal—they never die! Cancer cells divide and grow so rapidly that they form tumors. And they keep dividing and reproducing until they have completely taken over their host—the unfortunate individual with cancer.

Your cells are being constantly bombarded by chemicals, radiation, viruses and free-radical activity. Sooner or later, exposure to sunlight, chemicals or by-products from metabolizing your diet will damage one of the genes due to free-radical activity in your cell. A gene in your cell's DNA structure is damaged.

This cellular damage occurs in your body regularly during the millions of cell replacements that regeneration requires during your lifetime. Normally your body has powerful defenses in play to deal effectively with such damaged cells, expelling them from your system.

Eventually, however, it becomes increasingly difficult for your affected cells to maintain normal growth. That's because when the damaged DNA continually signals your body to grow and function, some genes get turned off that should be on, and vice versa. It is time for the body to defend itself against the invasion of this abnormal cell growth.

DNA-repair genes move into action. These special genes make proteins that correct the errors that occur whenever a cell copies its DNA during cell division. But if repair genes cannot do the job, then genetic mistakes continue to accumulate.

Tumor-suppressor genes are another line of defense. These important genes function to restrain cell growth and division. They try to control the abnormal growth of the damaged cells. When these tumor-suppressor genes are absent or become inactive, cells can begin to multiply out of control.

Still another line of defense involves the *growth genes* that regulate normal cell growth and division. If these genes get stuck in the "on" position, cell growth continues unhindered.[5]

A malignant appetite

Free from all the normal cellular restraints, the abnormal cells become malignant and begin to break all the rules. They divide uncontrollably, become less attached to their neighbors and invade space occupied by normal cells. These rapidly growing, out-of-control cells begin to burst out of the rank and file of normal cells and start creating tumors.

These renegade cells seem to take on a life of their own. To multiply as rapidly as they want to, they need an increased supply of blood. Through a process called "angiogenesis," malignant cells secrete chemicals that attract and promote the formation of new blood vessels. Now the tumor has its own steady supply of nutrients with which to feed itself; it can grow without any further limitations.

The tumor spreads through a process called "metastasis," in which a part of the tumor breaks off and migrates through the blood and lymphatic systems. Eventually the runaway cells colonize other parts of the body, creating even more tumors.[6] This is the end of the story of how a normal, healthy cell becomes a monstrous, murderous cancer cell.

Boveri wondered if cancer was caused by "growth stimulatory chromosomes." He speculated that some chromosomes had mysterious powers to make cells grow. He theorized that the unlimited, uncontrolled growth of tumors might be caused when a permanent increase in such cell matter was present.

Following the direction of his research, some scientists had embraced a new paradigm for defining the disease of cancer. Rather than calling cancer a "tumor," they understood that cancer was a *systemic disease*, of which a tumor was merely symptomatic. With that paradigm shift came the dramatic shift where to look for the causes and cure of the disease. Cancer researchers had begun to look for the cause of the systemic breakdown of the body's cellular health. With this new paradigm in place, they explained the cause of cancer as the body's turning on wild, out-of-control cellular growth. They became committed to learning how to help the body "turn off" this destructive process. Their search led them even deeper into the tiny world of DNA.

DNA and telomeres

In 1962, the Nobel Prize for Medicine was awarded to John Watson, Francis Crick and Maurice Wilkins for discovering the structure of DNA, the hereditary-containing substance found in cells. The applications of this remarkable discovery that defines an individual's characteristics are many.

One question the discovery of DNA provoked from biologists and other scientists was whether the body contained a biological clock that determines when a human being should begin to age. The research of Doctors Calvin Harley, Carol Greider and Bruce Futcher resulted in the discovery of a genetic mechanism in the cell that does function as a clock. The ticking of this clock depends on the length of *telomeres*, which are long threads carrying important genetic messages that cause the cells to regenerate.

They discovered that when a cell divides, it loses from five to twenty pieces of the telomeres. When all the segments of the telomeres are gone, the messages they convey are interrupted, and the cell stops regenerating itself. They concluded correctly that the length of these threads determines how long a cell family will live.[7]

It is considered a possibility that the shortening of the telomeres in cellular division may also contribute to the development of diseases such as arteriosclerosis, osteoarthritis, osteoporosis and diabetes. Scientists believe that if they can control this disintegration of the telomeres, aging could be delayed, and disease could be controlled at a cellular level.

Telomerase—a tail of time

Telomerase is an enzyme that rebuilds the body's telomeres as they continuously change in length. Scientists are particularly excited about the significance of telomerase to genetic cancer research because their tests have indicated that it may function in part to influence the longevity of a cell. When skin, retinal and vascular cells in the laboratory were triggered to produce telomerase, the internal clocks of these cells were rewound, and the cells lived much longer than normal.

These scientists believe they are the first to extend the life of human cells through these experiments. When cells were engineered to produce telomerase, which older cells do not do, they continued to divide rapidly.[8]

As we stated, cancer cells, unlike normal human cells, do not die. Instead, they replicate so rapidly that they form tumors. Scientists researching the enzyme telomerase also discovered that cancer cells contain telomerase. Researchers theorized that it was the telomerase in the cancer cells that caused them to keep replicating. Then scientists reasoned that if they could understand what causes cancer cells to live on endlessly, they could make some cellular adjustments that might force the cancer cells to die.

Further research has proven that tumors circumvent the natural life cycle of the cell both by inactivating the cell-death pathway and by switching on telomerase. This is the secret to the immortality of cancer cells. With the help of the enzyme telomerase, these renegade cells acquire the capacity for infinite cell division.[9] These important discoveries were unlocking the characteristics of cancer cells in such a way that scientists could begin to study ways to alter their behavior. Other breakthroughs would follow that would bring the reality of a cure much closer.

Oncogenes—cancer-causing genes

Our amazing prophet, Boveri, knew nothing of genes. However, if you substitute the word *gene* for *chromosome*, it would be fair to say that Boveri's genius predicted the Nobel-prize winning discovery of cellular "proto-oncogenes" by Harold Varmus and Mike Bishop in the 1970s.[10] These scientists were able to look deeper in the character of the human cell to prove what Boveri could only speculate, that some "chromosomes" had the powers to make cells grow.

These scientists discovered that an oncogene, a gene in a virus, gave a normal cell the ability to become malignant or cancerous. These genes are actually programmed to cause cancer. In addition to these genes that can cause cancer tumors to form, other genes exist that do just the opposite. Anti-oncogenes are genes that suppress or keep tumors from forming.

The discovery of this incredible genetic information has completely transformed cancer research. Varmus and Bishop proved that genes that are present in all normal living cells can actually change and become cancer cells. Any cell can become deregulated, amplified or overexpressed and thus contribute to malignancy.[11]

These two great scientists found that tumor viruses could make normal cells express the characteristic rapid, uncontrolled growth of cancerous cells. This was the breakthrough discovery for which Varmus and Bishop received the Nobel Prize. Scientists were thrilled, for cancer appeared to be giving up its secrets. They were beginning to unravel the mystery of cancer. If they could determine what "turned on" the rapid growth of cancer cells, they knew they were very close to developing methods to alter that activity, or "turn it off."

Mapping the human genome

Although the announcement of a cancer cure had proven to be premature, research scientists still believed they were pursuing the right course. They believed a cure for cancer could be discovered by understanding chromosomes and genes, their many functions and their amazing characteristics. It was here in this smallest picture of life that cancer cells were being programmed to spin out of control. Scientists believed they would find the information they needed here to reprogram the activity of these cells to develop a cure for cancer.

Techniques for studying the formation, function and structure of genes, called "cytogenetics," were developed. Scientific research became devoted to the careful study of the human *genome*. A genome is the complete set of chromosomes containing all the genetic information in your body. Science is getting increasingly closer to mapping the entire genetic physical "personality." Members of the scientific community concur that this achievement will be one of the greatest scientific accomplishments of all time. Understanding the human genome will help scientists better understand what can go wrong in the body and how to fix it.

Your genes are arranged in tightly coiled threads of DNA organized into pairs of chromosomes in most of your body's cells. You may know that genes can promote or cause disease when they don't work properly. Matt Ridley, head of the England-based International Centre, described a project dedicated to sequencing or mapping out the particular characteristics of each gene in a particular chromosome (called chromosome 22). According to Ridley, genome mapping is a way to decode all of human DNA. "The whole project once completed will be one of the most significant scientific achievements in all time," said Ridley. "It's the instruction manual for our species and the complete guide for how to build and run the human body."

Many scientists believe that one of the most powerful weapons in the fight against cancer is now within our grasp— the complete sequencing of human and mouse genomes. Our newly acquired ability to call up the entire array of genes and their sequences has already transformed our approaches to cancer genetics. This information is providing an armory of weapons in the war on cancer, one of which is the ability to create new drugs for specific types of cancer.

The Philadelphia Chromosome

The story of the Philadelphia chromosome classically illustrates how cancer drugs can be developed from an understanding of these genetic changes in cancer cells. The Philadelphia chromosome is a "broken" or malfunctioning chromosome found in chronic myeloid leukemia, a blood cancer with a particular cell type. It was first discovered in 1960.

It took more than a decade of research after its discovery to identify which chromosome was being altered when a portion of it was transferred to another chromosome. It took another ten years to learn which gene was activated as a result of this change. Even with this information, twenty more years of research were required to develop a drug that could specifically target the activated gene.[12]

Philadelphia chromosomes have been damaged during cell division and have become cancerous. The defective chromosomes had activated a gene that began programming the cells to grow out of control, causing malignancy. Researchers were able to identify exactly what mistake these cells were making that made them defective.

They were finally able to isolate the defect in the chromosomes and then isolate the gene that was activated to cause the cancer. Armed with this vital information, they could then find a drug to deactivate this cancer-producing gene. In other words, researchers developed a drug that could "turn off" this cancer at the gene level.

Many more of these studies have been conducted—especially for types of leukemia—that have identified a series of specific chromosomal changes associated with malignancy.[13]

Mutation point identified

Through this kind of dedicated research, the hidden, terrifyingly destructive world of cancer was finally being exposed. Scientists learned how to create cancer in a petri dish under the microscope. This visibility provided the first real demonstration of the causal role of genetic alterations in cell transformation.

The studies that followed had an electrifying effect on the field of cancer genetics. They showed it was possible to make a specific change in DNA, then transfer that altered DNA into a healthy cell, which would become cancerous. It was transferred in the form of a genome, as we have described—a complete set of chromosomes that contains the entire genetic information present in a cell.

As a result, the healthy cell began acting like a cancerous one. Through this technique researchers were discovering precisely why a particular cell breaks out from the rank and file and becomes a deadly killer.[14]

Additional research identified the exact point at which a mutation happened, causing a gene to become activated and breaking out to create cancer. This renegade gene is a proto-oncogene that scientists called HRAS. In further animal studies, case after case showed that this same gene was the one that was activated in animal cancers.[15]

What is really exciting is that these same genes were activated as a direct response to particular cancer-causing substances.[16] What a breakthrough! Now, a researcher could introduce a cancer-causing substance and watch to see which cells became renegade and turned cancerous. These amazing studies gave cancer researchers an understanding of the first direct link between exposure to cancer-causing materials and direct changes in genes that cause malignancies.[17]

Tumor-Suppressor Genes

As we have discussed, the decades of the 1970s and 1980s were filled with scientific research discoveries related to oncogenes. The 1990s would herald another startling breakthrough in the search for a cure for cancer: the discovery of the *tumor-suppressor gene*.

Tumor-suppressor genes are agents in the body that keep cells from forming cancer. These genes form a protective mechanism that helps to keep normal cells in check. Only when the protective force of these tumor-suppressor cells is minimized or blocked by outside forces do tumors become free to grow out of control.[18] Understanding what blocks the function of these suppressor genes would be a key to the coming cancer cure as well.

A predisposition for cancer?

The early pioneer Boveri had theorized that those who developed cancer might have an inherited predisposition to the disease based upon the lack or weakness of suppressor genes (chromosomes).[19] He went further to speculate, correctly, that for a cancer tumor to develop in this way, both parents would need to give their offspring a similar genetic weakness.[20] Boveri's theory provided a cellular explanation for the increased cancer rate in the children of cancer victims.

Research scientists throughout this century have realized that this inherited aspect of cancer held profound keys to the mystery of cancer, keys that could unlock even more doors to a coming cure. In 1971, A. G. Knudson conducted a study of a form of eye cancer in young children called "retinoblastoma." This cancer forms a tumor in the retina and is usually hereditary. Because of this hereditary nature, scientists believed it could reveal some vital information about how cancer is genetically inherited.

Knudson's studies echoed some of Boveri's predictions, but went farther in providing a mathematical formula of the probability of inheriting cancer from your parents. By inheriting two genetic factors, your own genetics could completely inactivate your body's natural tumor suppressors.[21]

Knudson's studies suggested that inheriting specific abnormalities or mutations in a suppressor gene is what predisposes you to cancer. Even with those inherited traits, developing cancer tumors required something more. Only when these cells with "weaker" genetic material reproduced abnormally could they become malignant.[22]

But what exactly were these abnormalities? Where were the particular tumor-suppressor genes located in a person's DNA? And how would knowing such information be helpful to finding a cancer cure? So much of cancer's mystery remained unsolved.

Knudson's theories of inherited predisposition for cancer needed to be tested. Another team of scientists, W. K. Cavenee and his colleagues, stepped onto the scene and added substance and credibility to Knudson's theories.[23] They created methods for tracking the parental origins of particular genes, including tumor suppressors. In so doing, they were able to witness the fate of these genes when cells made fatal mistakes during cell division resulting in cancer tumors. These tools were used to find the exact family of genes responsible for breast and colon cancers.[24] Tumor-suppressor genes (the RB gene) were mapped and cloned.[25]

Not only were the specific genes discovered for these cancers, which was a wonderful breakthrough in itself, but the pathways in which they assisted in the creation of cancer were also better understood. This knowledge is fueling the dream of scientists to one day create drugs to target specific genes to fight cancer or to strengthen genetic weaknesses providing a person's body with a better, stronger supply of tumor suppressors aimed like bullets at the bull's-eye where cancer forms.

Although these breakthrough scientific discoveries may seem complicated to the non-scientist, it is easy to understand that their implications are wonderfully far reaching. Researchers are actually looking deep inside the human mechanisms of life and, like genetic repairmen, are searching for ways to fix weak and broken

> **Exploration has already created a brave new world of cancer treatments that are filled with the promise of a coming cure.**

genetic material to halt cancer. Could scientists even a century ago have dreamed that such a thing was possible?

It is wonderful for the sake of understanding cancer that we are finding genetic weaknesses that may predispose people to it. I believe that these findings will help us develop promising therapeutic tools. However, I do not advise that you start finding an oncologist in your area just because there is "cancer in the family."

What these pioneering scientists are not clearly telling us is that the "bad genes," in order to do their mischievous deeds, need to be triggered and that "good genes" can be triggered to do bad deeds by the same triggers!

Consider the fact that American women have one of the highest rates of breast cancer in the world; surely the bad BRCA genes are running rampant in the United States. One the other hand, Chinese women have one of the lowest, if not the lowest, rates of breast cancer. Obviously they have been spared from the BRCA gene attack. Unfortunately, as soon as Chinese women

move to the United States and adopt the American way of eating, their rate of breast cancer evens up.

One genetic discovery opens vistas of other new possibilities
for the treatment and cure of cancer and other diseases.
Scientists have become explorers of microcosmic space in the
same way that our ancestors explored the macrocosmic spaces of
the earth and twenty-first-century astronauts explore the
expanses of the universe. Their exploration has already created a
brave new world of cancer treatments that are filled with promise
of a coming cure.

3 A Brave New World of Cancer Drugs

We are approaching the day when cancer patients will go to their doctors and, as routinely as they have been accustomed to giving blood samples, will give a sample of their DNA that will clinically map their entire human genome. Physicians will then be able to prescribe medicines according to the patient's precise weaknesses discovered in his or her DNA.

The wonder of DNA is that its spiraling strands resident in everyone's cells are not identical to the strands of any other person. These genetic instructions contain about three billion individualized molecules. Although 99.9 percent of those instructions may be the same for all individuals, that 0.1 percent of difference—about three million genes—contains our personal identity. These individual genes, called polymorphisms, program us to have different colored eyes and personal thumbprints, as well as a variety of personalized abilities.

Some day scientists hope to be able to catalog each person's thousands of genetic polymorphisms into a sort of genetic bar code. This bar code would be used to determine which drugs are safe for you to take and which ones could create adverse reactions because of your personal DNA. It will also tell your doctor the diseases to which you may be susceptible. At some point you will be able to get a genetic test to determine the cancers to which your body is predisposed.[1]

At least this is the new approach that cancer research scientists are pursuing. Such an approach promises to transform medicine. Already, pharmaceutical and biotech companies are investing millions of dollars to catalog and exploit human genetic differences to create a drug targeted to bring personalized healing.

"Precision" Cancer Drugs

A few years ago, Bob was lying on his back in a California hospital room wondering if he shouldn't just commit suicide and end it all. The pain in his bones caused by cancer was driving him crazy. Even the slightest movement sent pain screaming through his body. To get to the bathroom, he was reduced to crawling across the floor on his knees. Pain, humiliation and hopelessness flooded his mind and body.

Instead of pursuing thoughts of self-destruction, Bob decided to enter an experimental program for a new cancer drug. The results of this drug therapy were nothing short of miraculous. Bob soon returned to normal life and was able to go back to work. He reported, "I go to the gym. I have a girlfriend. It's the dream of any cancer patient in the world to be able to take a pill that works like this. It's truly a miracle."[2]

In 1999, a New York cancer patient, Victoria, believed she had only a few months remaining to live. She was suffering from chronic myeloid leukemia, a deadly type of blood cancer. The only treatment available for this kind of cancer made her deathly ill and was not really working. She spent most of her time in bed for a year, too sick to walk or even lie in bed and read.

Victoria also joined an experimental program for a new cancer drug. Within weeks after beginning her drug therapy everything changed for her—suddenly she could read and take a walk. Before the year was over, clinical tests showed that Victoria's bone marrow was free of leukemia cells. By the New Year, she had signed up for dancing lessons.[3]

～

For Bob and Victoria there were no cancerous tumors to excise. Their "miraculous" cures were a result of years of research based on an entirely new approach to treating cancer. Attacking these forms of cancer required oncologists to make a dramatic shift from the "cancer is a tumor" paradigm. To conquer cancer, researchers had begun to realize they needed a better understanding of this complicated disease.

Aside from surgery, which almost invariably leaves behind some malignant cells, standard treatment for most cancers continues to be radiation and chemotherapy. Clinical studies continue to show that these are relatively crude disease-fighting weapons with limited effectiveness. They bring with them terrible side effects that weaken a patient and compromise his or her immune system.

Some researchers believe the results of the standard treatments for cancer are unacceptable. They continue to work to solve the mystery of how cancer works at a molecular level—from its first breaking out of the rank and file of healthy DNA to its final destructive attack on the body. To them we owe the wonderful hope for the coming cure that is already making a difference for cancer patients like Bob and Victoria.

Using the wealth of knowledge they have already gained, scientists have developed precision cancer-fighting drugs designed to halt and block the disease at every step. Unlike chemotherapy and radiation that indiscriminately attack all the body's cells, both good and bad, these new cancer drugs will attack cancer at the precise point of cellular breakdown causing the disease. These new cancer strategies find the weakest link predisposed to disease and eliminate it.

One of cancer's weakest links is called *growth factors*. These growth factors form an entire class of biological signals that aid and assist cancer cells to grow out of control. Scientists are working hard to find ways to halt the destructive work of these growth factors. Another "weak link" or destructive characteristic of cancer cells, as we have mentioned, is their immortality—they refuse to die. Scientists are developing drug therapies also that will program cancer cells to self-destruct.

Still other therapies will block enzymes that cancer cells use to chew openings in normal tissues, thereby giving them room to expand. And *angiogenesis inhibitors*, one of the most celebrated brave new approaches to cancer treatment, are powerful compounds that will keep tumors from building new blood vessels that aid their growth by supplying them with food and oxygen.

Magic Bullets?

Though these scientific wonders are on the horizon, we must not raise our expectations too high too soon. They are not magic bullets. It is uncertain how many years will be required to complete all the studies and discover all the means necessary to reach those goals. In the meantime, step by step, through the efforts of modern cancer research, we are making progress against this disease.

Many of the treatments being explored today do not have as their goal a complete cure for cancer. Instead, the goal of these treatments is to hinder and slow the progress of the dreaded disease, transforming it into a much more manageable enemy. Experts hope they can tame this deadly disease through treatment, as has been done with diabetes and high blood pressure.

Drug treatments that can lessen the impact of cancer, making it a chronic disease that does not result in death, will represent progress toward a complete cure. And it will have great impact on the improved quality of life for cancer patients. We must, however, underscore the need for individualized treatment and the use of great caution in applying these new drug therapies. Rob's story dramatically illustrates this serious concern.

Rob was a nine-year-old boy who was near death when he

arrived at Mayo Clinic. He had been battling leukemia for quite some time, but that's not the reason he was critically ill. To treat his leukemia, Rob had been given thiopurine drug. This kind of drug has been known to transform acute lymphoblastic leukemia—previously considered a virtual death sentence—into a disease which has an 80 percent survival rate.

Unfortunately, one in three hundred Caucasians possess a genetic makeup that alters the drug's action in the body. Instead of fighting the leukemia in these patients, the drug destroys bone marrow. Rob was one of those rare patients. His story ended well, however. Under the care of the Mayo doctors, his bone marrow slowly recovered from the ill effects of the drug, and in three months he was able to go home.[4]

When it comes to prescribing a new drug therapy for the treatment of cancer, doctors must be keenly aware that there are no magic bullets. This fact has spurred researchers on to determine healing solutions for the kind of exception Rob was. In 1991, researchers perfected a simple way to test for the genetic variation shared by this boy. Today, medical centers routinely test for it and tailor their drug treatments accordingly.

This child's story underscores the incredible promise of genetically tailored treatments. It also warns of the treacherous mountains that must be scaled in a new frontier of personally tailored medical treatments.

Pros and Cons of Drug Therapies

As responsible physicians, we must be realistic when considering the use of cancer drug therapies, no matter the hype that surrounds them. While we cannot afford to ignore such promising therapies, we must also be aware of the downside of their use, which includes their exorbitant cost, limited success rates and possible side effects. Given those cautions, we can consider their positive treatment value for each individual patient.

For example, researchers discovered some time ago that cancer cells rely upon an unusually large number of proteins that make up each cell. These proteins provide receptacles for fuel, including the fuel provided by growth factors. Therefore, scientists determined that if they could target these proteins—or more precisely the receptors housed by them—they could send ammunition to where it would do the most damage.

They developed a drug called *Rituxan* (manufactured by Genentech/IDEC) that is a monoclonal antibody specifically engineered to fit into the receptacles on non-Hodgkin's lymphoma cells and single out cancer cells for destruction by the immune system. However, in the 1980s, monoclonal antibodies were too optimistically heralded as the magic bullets that would wipe out cancer completely.[5] The medical community is sadder but wiser now.

Another consideration for the use of this drug is the cost. A four-week treatment with Rituxan costs $10,000 to $20,000, which is prohibitive for some patients. In addition, it is not without side effects. Those taking this treatment can expect to experience fever, chills and in rare cases low blood pressure and potentially fatal allergic reactions.[6]

Growth factor inhibitors

Herceptin, a breast cancer drug manufactured by Genentech, uses the same approach as Rituxan to fight cancer. The difference between them is that where Rituxan carefully targets cancer cells for destruction, Herceptin targets specific cancer cells to keep them from growing. It keeps growth factors from feeding and nourishing certain kinds of breast cancer cells. The total cost of the thirty-six-week treatment is about $25,000. And its side effects are similar to Rituxan, in that it causes fever, chills and in rare cases heart problems and potentially fatal allergic reactions.[7]

For drugs like Herceptin to work effectively, a patient's cancer must have ample receptor sites to which it can attach. Herceptin latches onto a receptor known as HER2, which is found in abnormally large amounts in nearly a third of all breast cancers. If an individual's cancer is not rich in these receptors, it will not respond to the drug.

Dr. John Mendelsohn, president of the M. D. Anderson Cancer Center in Houston, had been looking for other receptor sites that would serve the same purpose. Since 1981 he has been studying a close cousin of receptor HER2 called EGFR, which is host to a protein called epidermal growth factor (EGF). Nearly two-thirds of all cancer types are blanketed with EGF receptors.

In 1984, Mendelsohn and his team were able to block this receptor with a growth-factor decoy that stopped the cancer cell from growing and dividing.[8] Here is the trick: Receptors like HER2 also show up in normal cells. Nevertheless, researchers have learned that normal cells are more adept than cancer cells at finding other receptor cells to rely on when EGFR is blocked.

Recently, Mendelsohn revealed a drug compound called IMC-C225, which was proven to be effective in treating a small number of colon cancer patients.[9] When this drug is combined with more traditional colorectal chemotherapy treatments, researchers at Sloan-Kettering saw cancer tumors shrink in 20 percent of otherwise hopeless cases. It is believed that the growth-factor inhibitor is weakening the tumors enough for chemotherapy to then come in and finish them off.[10]

Other experimental drugs, such as Gleevec, are designed on the same growth-inhibiting principle. Gleevec was responsible for the dramatic recovery of the leukemia patient we met earlier. Another growth-inhibiting drug is Tarceva, a drug from OSI Pharmaceuticals that shows promise against some lung cancer tumors and head and neck cancers. Neither of these preparations prevents EGF from docking with cells. Instead, they make their way inside the cells, intercepting growth messages.

Herceptin, Gleevec and the other hopeful new drug therapies represent an entirely new generation of cancer treatments that target the biological signals that promote cancer-cell growth.

Forcing cancer cells to die

Other drug therapies are targeting the immortality of the cancer cell. As we've discussed, cancer cells don't die. While all of our body's normal cells know when their life cycle is over, cancer cells do not. Left unchecked, they keep growing, dividing and multiplying until they have destroyed everything healthy and normal in their path.

One new treatment is looking at the possibility of outsmarting this perpetual growth pattern from inside the cell. Scientists are looking at a group of enzymes called *caspaces*. They are experimenting to see if blocking these enzymes could keep DNA from repairing their cell's telomeres each time they divide.[11] Remember that every time a normal cell divides, their telomeres (a cell's biological clock) become shorter. When a telomere is used up, the cell dies. Cancer cells have a telomere repair mechanism that perpetuates their existence.

LDP341 is a proteasome-inhibiting substance that interferes with the telomere repairing capacity of the malignant cell. Scientists hope that this and other similar substances could shorten the life span of a malignant cell. I would be generous and give them a few minutes, even days. Proteasome is a protein that has a role in cancer's longevity. Studies by Millennium Pharmaceuticals in Massachusetts seem promising.

Cutting off blood supply

Pioneering research for drugs that could cut off the blood supply to cancerous tumors began in the 1970s when overzealous and over-optimistic researchers thought these drugs would provide the entire answer for curing cancer, not just a part of it. They were still functioning under the "cancer is a tumor" paradigm, which led them to believe if they could starve the tumor they could cure cancer.

It is true that every organ and tissue in your body must have some kind of supporting blood supply to give it oxygen and nourishment. Invading cancer tumors are no different.

Therefore, reversing this principle to keep a tumor from getting the nourishment it needs is an effective strategy for the promising *antiangiogenesis* drugs.

A tumor seeks to find the blood supply it needs by first eating its way through healthy surrounding tissue to tap into blood vessels that contain the oxygen and nutrients it needs to survive. Eventually, the tumor has increased so much that it has the power to begin growing its own capillaries and blood vessels.[12]

The work of the antiangiogenesis drugs is to cut off the blood supply to the tumor, which will slow its growth. Although the results have been wonderful in mice, researchers aren't seeing the same success in humans. Only a tiny number of human subjects treated with these preparations have seen their tumors shrink. Nevertheless, researchers remain very hopeful. Even though antiangiogenesis drugs do not seem to be making cancer go away, they do effectively slow its growth.[13] Clinicians believe that these preparations can become a vital part of a larger chemical cocktail that will be able to attack and destroy cancer using several of the above strategies at a time.

Questions to Be Answered

A decade ago, there were one hundred twenty-four medicines in the research pipeline being tested as potential anticancer drugs. Today there more than four hundred, and the list is growing. (Please see Appendix A for further discussion of some of the most common cancer drugs.) As promising as these cancer drugs are, many questions remain to be answered before they can be a more effective part of the coming cure for cancer.

Among the most important questions to be answered is, *Which patient needs which drug?* The goal of cancer researchers is to be able to detect precisely which molecular processes have gone wrong in each person who is a victim of cancer. Rather than the disease being classified as lung or liver or colon cancer, it will be classified according to the genetic abnormality that triggered it, such as "EGFR positive."

The dream of these scientists is to be able to say one day to Mrs. Smith, who has breast cancer, "There are four genes that are abnormal in your tumor." Then her doctor will open a drawer and choose the antibodies or small molecules designed to attack the abnormal products of those genes. He can then give her a cocktail targeting the genes that caused her cancer and expect her to be cured.

The excitement of this dream quickly dwindles when you move from the confines of the wishful world of research and face desperation in the most real arena of daily medical practice. Our patients' patience is amazing, but often, too often, time will not be on their side. To the person put on death row by a no-nonsense tumor, the brilliant (but distant) future of research provides little solace.

So many faces constantly flash through my mind. There is the fragile, loving face of Amy, a ten-year-old girl from Australia. Her lovely face had lost its beauty due to the growth of a tumor in her mouth that could not be stopped in spite of all the orthodox and unorthodox therapies she received. She died in her mother's arms after a valiant fight. It is in these painful moments of loss that the advances of science seem so vain, so terribly empty.

Yet, it is because of the Amys of the world that we must persist in our quest to eradicate the *terror* of cancer. I choose my words carefully, even respectfully, since cancer is a monumental adversary. Completely eradicating this terrorist disease may only happen in the distant future. But eradicating the *terror* this disease provokes is, as we will see, a reachable goal in our time.

It may seem unfair that the hope of eradicating cancer, so real and attainable, will be enjoyed by future generations while we continue to be ravaged by the disease. But this has been the experience of past generations also who suffered diseases that we have since eradicated. How many died, for instance, of childbirth until research discovered the effectiveness of birth by C-section? And deadly infections that killed people by the millions in the past are now a medical "child's game," thanks to pharmaceutical developments brought about by research. Unfortunately, research does not come cheap.

"Uhh...your bill, Mrs. Smith!"

That dream is sure to come at a high price. The drug of choice for Mrs. Smith's breast cancer could cost her as much as $2,500 per month for the rest of her life. While the National Cancer Institute funds basic research into cancer biology, the bulk of cancer drugs are developed by for-profit pharmaceutical firms. Such firms claim that it costs them between $500 million and $1 billion to bring a single new cancer drug to consumers. That fact makes cancer *big business*, which is an important aspect of cancer treatment to consider when you are choosing your personal therapy.

4 Caution: Following the Money Trail

In our hospital, The Oasis of Hope, in Tijuana, Mexico, we have marveled at the benefits of the advances medical science is making in so many ways. We witnessed some of these benefits to one of our colleagues in a special way when he suffered a tragic accident several years ago.

Francisco Bucio, M.D., one of our plastic surgeons, was working in a hospital in Mexico City when the devastating earthquake of 1985 struck that city. As he was making his customary rounds, the hospital collapsed around him during that earthquake. When Dr. Bucio was rescued from the rubble and debris sometime later, four fingers on his right hand were completely crushed. Those fingers had to be amputated, leaving only his thumb. You can imagine the devastating tragedy this would be for a surgeon whose hands are so vital to his vocation.

Although he was convinced that his career as a surgeon was over, Dr. Bucio decided to submit to surgery performed by a fellow plastic surgeon from the United States. The surgeon transposed two of Dr. Bucio's toes, the longest from each foot, attaching them to his hand. He now has opposing "fingers" to the thumb, which form a functional hand. Isn't that unbelievable? But that's not the end of the story.

Today he is one of the busiest plastic surgeons in our city due to his excellent abilities. Now, that's what I call a miracle! Yes, medicine has come a long way, and at times its advances leave us awe-struck.

Scientists claim that in a couple of decades, knowledge obtained from the human genome will enable geneticists to "direct" DNA information to specific areas to rebuild body parts, like the lizards that grow their cutoff tails. Even if it would take Dr. Bucio years to retrain a genetically grown hand, I believe he would be thrilled with the possibility. Many people are being helped in fantastic ways because of the explosion of technology in the last few years. Unfortunately, these technological successes are not the entire story.

A Technological Explosion

The second half of the twentieth century boasted the greatest technological explosion in the history of medicine. Genetic engineering, chemical syntheses of pharmaceuticals, computerization in microbiology, nuclear medicine, gamma knife, transplants, endoscopic surgery, surgical training simulators and hundreds of other genuinely amazing scientific advances contributed to that explosion.

And in the clinical field, new devices greatly facilitate the work of physicians. Now there are computer programs that can diagnose and recommend a treatment. It is possible to examine organs using a tiny probe that functions as a video camera instead of the more invasive approach that surgery required. Accident victims can now be attended to rapidly by teams of highly trained doctors, nurses and technicians that often bring patients "back" to life.

Nowhere is the stunning prowess of modern medicine so readily displayed as it is in the area of cancer research. We have already discussed some of the wonderful breakthroughs this research has achieved. The American medical machine that drives this research is the most powerful in the world. And its engine devoted to cancer research is no less dazzling.

Billions of dollars have been invested into medical science

during the twentieth century to make its remarkable achievements possible. It is this fact, the high cost of researching, developing and marketing these therapies, drugs and equipment, that begs the question: From where does all of this money come? And, more importantly, how do such massive amounts of money impact the quality, availability and objectivity of medical services and products? Can such huge amounts of cash cloud the medical community's ability to do what is best for those suffering with cancer and other diseases?

It is important to understand the money question lurking behind the medical industry's achievements. Though it may seem that the subject of "big business" in the world of medical science is as cold and impersonal as a doctor's stethoscope, it could become as personal an issue as your choice of a therapy for a life-threatening disease. Experience has taught us that the pathway to the truth of any issue never lies far from the money trail.

Beginnings of the
Modern Medical Machine

It may be surprising to some to learn that it was not until after the turn of the twentieth century that the first pharmaceutical drugs were mass-produced and marketed. It is disconcerting to many of us that the first drugs produced were involved in a controversy as to the benefit to the patient vs. monetary gain.

Paul Ehrlich, considered the father of the pharmaceutical industry, was the first person to produce pharmaceuticals in an organized way. He received a Nobel Prize in 1908 for developing an effective drug to treat syphilis. The compound he developed was known as the "magic bullet" *Salvarsan*. The treatment—used throughout Europe and America under the name *Triparsamide*—was first produced by Merck Laboratories. And the American Medical Association (AMA) backed and promoted its massive distribution

Even from its humble beginnings, the priorities of the pharmaceutical industry have been somewhat less than altruistic.

Business and financial concerns were a part of the "mother's milk" shortly after the birth of the industry. Ehrlich's drug for syphilis was produced and distributed with the blessing of the AMA even after Dr. Ehrlich recommended that it be abandoned because he had learned that it caused blindness.

Some years later in 1928, Alexander Fleming accidentally discovered penicillin. Fleming had been engaged in the search for causative agents in the influenza epidemic of 1918, which killed twenty-five million people. Rushing to leave on holiday, he accidentally left his bacterial cultures on a worktable in his London laboratory.

While he was away, the cultures became contaminated with green fungus that succeeded in destroying the disease-causing microorganisms of the culture. Of course, the green fungus contained what is now known as penicillin, which became one of the standard antibiotics of this century. Fleming's fortuitous oversight merited him the 1945 Nobel Prize for the discovery of penicillin.

With the discovery of penicillin, the mass production of antibiotics began. Since that time medicine has not looked back. From the beginning, there has been a desire in the medical science community to find a "magic bullet"—one pill or medication that will stop the pain and destroy the disease.

The Pharmaceutical Industry: Big Business

The modern medical establishment was birthed in the pangs of plagues, disease and pestilence, which raged through European towns and ravaged entire populations. A terrifying death toll was exacted upon our ancestors during these plagues of Europe. Since then, the improvement of health worldwide has been attributed to the development of drugs and vaccines that destroy germs and disease-causing agents.

However, little is mentioned concerning the fact that the deplorable conditions of filth and stench in which these suffering populations lived have also been eliminated. It is almost inconceivable for those of us living in Western cultures today to imagine the deplorable living conditions of those faraway times The plagues of Europe began to abate simultaneously as sanitary conditions, hygiene methods, better food distribution and city planning cleansed the environment in which the general population lived.

Two important innovations—appropriate management of sewage in the eighteenth century and the practice of quarantine—also yielded impressive results for the health of the general public. Yet the credibility and status of drugs and vaccines grew to mammoth proportions during these formative years of the pharmaceutical industry. Their celebrated status shaped the worldwide mentality toward medical science and predisposed the world community to accept almost without question the solutions it offered.

Guidelines for pharmaceuticals

From the infancy of the pharmaceutical industry, governments realized they needed to establish and maintain strict guidelines for the production and distribution of pharmaceuticals in order to protect consumers. Controlling the manufacturing process of pharmaceuticals is vitally important because they are potentially dangerous.

Throughout the world, governmental authorities "look out" for the interests and health of their citizens. In many countries, public health departments require laboratories to adhere to ever-changing safety guidelines to market their products. Pharmaceutical laboratories are assigned registration numbers and licenses to produce, distribute and sell only drugs that are proven to be safe and effective. And these restrictions have been modified to become increasingly sophisticated, complicated and fantastically expensive.

Unfortunately, those authorities that are empowered to determine when and how these drugs will be delivered to the ill have many political voices vying for their ear. They are not always listening solely to the desperate patient, the family member or other consumer. The sound of the gentle voice of the patient and his or her family is often muffled by the booming voice of the financial investor.

The billions of dollars required to bankroll the testing, developing and marketing of drugs must be financed by someone. Wealthy investors in pharmaceutical companies keep a watchful eye on the earnings of their hefty ventures. Millions of dollars are lost when a particular drug doesn't pan out and fails to be approved. That loss is factored into the cost of the far fewer drugs that are approved.

As we have stated, drug companies claim it costs them between $500 million and $1 billion to bring a single new medicine to market. For every one drug approved by the FDA, five thousand others have failed. The drug companies count on that one success to pay for the five thousand failures.[1] Pharmaceutical patent-holders are given a monopoly on their particular drug for seventeen years to allow them to recoup their hefty investments.

There are other influential voices that try to be heard above that of the patient. The voices of those who produce scientific equipment, the distributors and others whose livelihood depends on the production of pharmaceuticals also worry about their share of the profits. This fact places the "well-being" of the patient far down the list of priorities for developing and marketing effective, reasonably priced drugs.

Afflictions or marketing opportunities?

Weighty financial pressures, those hefty costs of bringing a drug to the patients, force the pharmaceutical industry to deal with diseases more as marketing opportunities rather than as afflictions. The money trail continues to play a dramatic role in how fast research develops in a particular area.

For example, the AIDS virus has gained a powerful voice with governments, the FDA and pharmaceutical companies because of the overwhelming plague it has become with global consequences. Besides financial pressures that drive the pharmaceutical markets, there are other strong interests that make their voices heard. In the case of the terrible epidemic of AIDS, the voices of thousands of "activist" patients have influenced the FDA more than those with other life-threatening diseases. Research and development of treatments for AIDS have experienced far less resistance from the FDA to "short cut" their regulations for treatments because of the enormous pressure patients and activists have placed upon the U.S. government to find a cure.

In 1985, the National Institutes of Health (NIH) invited Burrows-Welcome, a British company with experience in antivirals (owners of the patent for the popular anti-flu Sudafed), to develop and manufacture a treatment against the AIDS plague. Researchers for the laboratory dug into the archives of their pharmacological junkyard and found an anticancer drug called AZT known for its antiviral properties and recommended its use to treat the AIDS virus.

Twenty-three years earlier, the FDA had rejected AZT as being primitive and extremely toxic. But the NIH caved in to the "pressure" of the AIDS epidemic and permitted its clinical application. They now determined the risks were acceptable because AIDS patients were sentenced to die from the disease.[2]

Losing no time, Burrows-Welcome presented their toxic drug to the establishment and requested a patent, which was granted in 1988. By 1992, the sales of AZT topped $100 million thanks to the sales pitch based on its temporary benefits. Investors enjoyed yet another financial success through the production of this pharmaceutical.[3] (For more discussion of the AIDS dilemma, please see Appendix B.)

This justification for use of a previously condemned drug may seem reasonable in the face of the present AIDS crisis. However, the same argument could be brought to bear from the nearly six hundred thousand cancer patients who face the same fatal prognosis each year. Yet, those sentenced to die of cancer receive no similar special status from the FDA. No "short cuts" are allowed to developing drug regulations that offer such alternatives for patients in the arena of cancer research!

Priority Conflicts

The AZT controversy epitomizes the circus of interests beyond humanitarianism that impact drug development and sales. Health departments, both here and abroad, are pillars of the global community entrusted with guardianship of public health. However, these pillars appear to bend under the pressure of political and financial interests. If such is the case, can we be certain that their top priority is to protect us from toxic or ineffective pharmaceuticals? Our very lives depend upon the answer to that question.

Health departments never conduct their own clinical studies. They simply approve or reject a drug on the basis of scientific research by the pharmaceutical industry. Effectiveness of a particular drug is determined by weighing the benefits of the treatment against the undesirable side effects. Therefore, if a few thousand patients suffer or die, those lives are expendable for the sake of the good experienced by others. Health departments have to make these terrible judgments on each therapy presented to them. And regardless of whose life is expended, the pharmaceutical laboratories get rich from marketing their product.

Lost objectivity

Pharmaceutical firms do not deny that most research for new drugs is done in-house, which has the potential for clouding the objectivity of these for-profit firms. They do involve independent institutions in their research, such as universities, that "impartially" corroborate their findings. These impartial studies are intended to give credibility to the more subjective findings of the pharmaceutical companies.

It is generally accepted that universities carry out their research in an unbiased manner. Supposedly they don't allow themselves to be influenced by the economic incentives they receive for their research, officially called "donations" and "scholarships," from the pharmaceutical industry. Yet, one wonders if the prospect of losing such subsidies could ever influence a university's or research group's findings on a drug or product.

Published and patented

I love research, and it has given me great satisfaction to publish nine articles in Austrian, German, Mexican and American medical journals. This accomplishment alone catapulted me to a higher echelon in the scientific hierarchy. It also taught me the valuable lesson that it is easy to get trapped in the web of "publicationism."

Academic researchers first engage in research for the sheer love of it. But too often they end up feeling the pressure to publish. In the scientific world, we call it the *publish-or-perish* mentality. Publication is the oxygen that researchers breathe. Their research conducted through long hours spent in isolated laboratories can eventually provide a vehicle for gaining instant acclaim and wide recognition among their peers.

And these publications can lead to more important achievements—patented rights. Industrial researchers are not motivated by this pressure of publicationism. Their motivation is purely and simply commercial advantage. The financial future of pharmaceuticals depends on the outcome of their research. Incentives for scientists at important universities like Harvard, MIT and Yale include being published in prestigious publications and receiving international recognition, scholarships and patent rights.

Patent rights given for credible scientific breakthroughs can generate wealth, power and the ultimate symbol of success—a Nobel Prize. Universities benefit greatly from their students' achievements. To support their efforts, universities provide their researchers with super laboratories and the assistance of the most promising students.

These prizes, medallions and remuneration possibilities are irresistible to scientists. Yet, human lives, the real object of research, lie in the balance. With so many pressures to succeed and so many tempting promises offered, can you imagine that purely altruistic motivation is ever swept aside in the laboratory?

How can government agencies protect us from dangerous medications if they depend on research conducted by a pharmaceutical industry that has sold out to fame and fortune? The coming cancer cure depends in part on the answer to this ethical question. As long as cancer research and pharmaceuticals are a part of big business, eradicating cancer will not be the priority it needs to be. Yet, the culture that this big business has spawned places more and more confidence in the latest drug produced. So business is good—but where are the cures? (Please see Appendix C for further discussion of these big business practices.)

Where are the modern scientists who are willing to put all their effort into serving humanity without regard to monetary gain and prestigious rewards? If the ultimate goal of medical science were to heal the sick, more scientists would behave like Dr. Jonas Salk, who developed the polio vaccine. Against the advice of his coworkers, he refused to patent his vaccine. He wanted the whole world to own it so that polio could be eradicated.[4]

Consequences of a "drug" culture

The words of Linnaeus in his eighteenth-century *Diaeta Naturalis (Natural Diet)* ring true: "To live dependent on medicine is to live hideously." His words have never taken on such depth of meaning until now, when so many people suffer from one disease or another and depend upon one or more medications to keep them going each day.

The most often prescribed drugs include tranquilizers, sleeping pills, high blood pressure drugs, arthritic painkillers and antibiotics. All of these are consumed in industrial-strength quantities. The size and scope of the pharmaceutical industry are at staggering proportions. Billions of these pills are sold annually by drugstores and consumed as a matter of habit by the average person. We must wonder what overall health effects our drug-dependent culture will experience and how it might impact future generations.

Although most of the information is not within the reach of the general public, records indicate there have been some tragic consequences for those charged with keeping watch over public health—especially the FDA—as a result of the prolific production of new drugs and therapies. Ill-fated drugs that they have approved for public consumption have damaged and destroyed hundreds of lives before their danger was detected.

The famous thalidomide incident is probably the worst such example. Ingested by pregnant women to combat nausea, it produced severe deformities in their offspring. Around fifteen hundred babies suffered the miserable consequences.[5] (Please see Appendix D for further discussion of some of these ill-fated drugs.)

A trail of broken promises

There is little doubt that cancer is the greatest challenge medical science has ever faced. No other disease has been given more money or more scientific hours of study. The sums devoted to looking for a cure could have bankrolled a small- to medium-sized country. Yet, even in today's prolific drug culture and progressive therapies, the promise of a "magic bullet" to cure cancer has continued to elude us.

In 1955, NCI established the Chemotherapy National Service Center (CNSC), appropriating $25 million to promote this anticancer treatment, since "it was demonstrated" that chemotherapy had "proved to be an effective treatment for cancer patients, not only in the United States, but around the world."[6] Why was so much money needed to promote an "effective" treatment?

Two years later Lawrence Rockafeller reported that oncological research was nearing a victory. "There is for the first time the smell of victory in the air," he said.[7]

For centuries, we have put our faith in doctors and the promised cures of medical science. Should we really put ourselves blindly into their hands? The confidence we have given to medical science has its roots in the conviction that research is carried out objectively in university and governmental institutions unencumbered by economic and political interests. We have believed that their discoveries and advances are motivated by a genuine concern for social well-being—and nothing else.

In this new millennium, the American Cancer Society predicts that 50 percent of men and 30 percent of women will develop some form of cancer in their lifetimes.[8] In May of 1986, Dr. John C. Bailar III of Harvard University and Elaine Smith of the University of Iowa published in the *New England Journal of Medicine* an "atomic bomb" against orthodox oncology. They concluded that the advances left much to be desired in view of the fact that the most common forms of cancer remained uncontrollable. They insisted that the scientific world reconsider the present guiding principles of cancer research, along with their application.

What's Wrong With This Picture?

A depressing picture of "approved" treatments against cancer, such as surgery, radiation and chemotherapy, is revealed in an evaluation made by the American Cancer Society. In its annual publication of *Cancer Facts and Figures* for 2001, all cancer rate improvements can be accounted for by a decline in the numbers of cigarette smokers and increased concern regarding diet and lifestyle, not from orthodox treatments.[9]

In most malignancies graphed, statistical records indicate that the "enormous scientific advances" have not helped patients survive. On the contrary, where the malignancies are treated with aggressive remedies, the death rates remain incredibly high. The death rate of people suffering from lung (pulmonary) cancer remains by far the highest, although it has experienced a modest decline that corresponds to the drop in smoking. Sadly, lung cancer is the number one killer in women as well as in men!

Despite all the promises and vast sums of research money poured into it, the treatment of cancer has really changed very little. Technological developments have been applied to these treatments, but technology has only served as a cosmetic improvement. In the meantime, we continue to fight cancer with the same weapons of surgery, radiation and chemotherapy, although with more sophisticated equipment and techniques. The medical community continues to redeal the same cards over and over again.

After watching the scientific community spend exorbitant amounts on an unsuccessful thirty-year research project to find a cure, I have come to conclude that prevention is the best medicine. But, where's the budget for prevention research?

The science of sabotage

In other branches of modern science and industry, obsolescence is an everyday occurrence that allows new processes to replace the old even if the old are still working. That has not been the case with the cancer issue. Regarding this life-threatening health issue, governmental authorities, the scientific community and pharmaceutical monopolies have refused to accept new ideas and new approaches to treatment of the disease.

Many promising alternative therapies for cancer, some of which have been proven effective, have been ridiculed, pushed aside and even prohibited by the above agencies. Even though these alternative therapies do not deteriorate the patients' quality of life, which is many times the case with orthodox treatments such as surgery and chemotherapy, they are not approved or promoted by the medical community.

The achievement that must truly be credited to the American medical industry is the creation of an omnipotent medical marketing machine. It has completely convinced doctors everywhere that America has divine knowledge and that all other medical communities should strive to be like its doctors.

The super technology and super specialties make a doctor feel like Superman. As a result, surgeons move faster than a speeding bullet to get more patients on the operating table. Yes, the medical establishment is stronger than a locomotive, but I fear that its patients are tied down to the train tracks. It is easy to run over your patients once you have dehumanized them by forgetting about the person and focusing only on the disease. In this regard, very little has changed since the early days of research when doctors viewed cancer as a "tumor" and its eradication was more important than extending the life of the patient.

Regard for the human touch

While the medical industry can boast of the might of its industrial machine, the downside of the industry is its glaring inability to recapture the human touch. The reading of the Hippocratic Oath still brings tears to the eyes of many doctors. And I believe there still exist altruistic humans behind cold stethoscopes. However, the pressures to keep up with overwhelming medical information, the costs of malpractice insurance and the stress of dealing with the sick and the dying make it almost "necessary" for doctors to detach their feelings from their patients.

And then, there is the issue of "medical" correctness. Modern doctors make every effort to avoid giving "false hope" to patients diagnosed with cancer. This practice often destroys whatever emotional fortitude a patient may have when faced with the life-threatening diagnosis. "If you do not start chemotherapy right away," the doctor tells the patient, "you will die within three months."

The trembling patient then asks, "Will the chemo get rid of it?"

"No, but it will give you maybe a year, enough time for you to get your affairs in order."

If the patient starts bargaining with proactive ideas, like changes in diet or taking vitamins, the oncologist will quell their enthusiasm with scientific terminalism, encouraging them to accept and understand the fact that the fight is futile.

No wonder the war against cancer is a failure; it neutralizes one of the most powerful weapons for survival—the courage and hope of the human psyche. If military generals "encouraged" their soldiers the way oncologists encourage their patients, all wars would have been lost!

Some of the most amazing speeches have been delivered to soldiers on the brink of battle. Has anyone accused Churchill or Patton of giving false hope to the soldiers that saved the world from Hitler? Their powerful words helped soldiers face bullets and bombs. For the survivors those words helped to keep them alive; for the fallen those same words gave them immortal honor.

Leadership is powerful; it is the driving force of purpose and hope that makes people willing to follow their leaders. And hope is a vital ingredient to bring life to any situation. Doctors need to understand the power of leadership and ways they can infuse life-threatening situations with hope. Confronted with a life-and-death crisis, a true leader inspires his soldiers with expectations for life.

Instead, oncologists typically lead their patients into expectations for accepting death as the only end. There is something wrong with this picture. Even if death is probable, a doctor should be able to help the patient live the rest of his shortened life with courage. And then he or she should help them look beyond death to the transcendence of eternal life.

If hope of surviving cancer can lead to success in life, what could lead to success beyond life? What transcends it? Not physical or emotional aptitudes; only spiritual forces and God provide solace in such an arena. However, physicians are convinced that they would transgress some hidden law if they touch this arena. I challenge this position. The human touch should necessarily include using our leadership role to give hope for life—here and beyond. Otherwise how can we, our patients and their loved ones cope with our tremendous limitations?

Technological achievements undeniably represent a huge

advance in the diagnosis and treatment of diseases. But no appa-
ratus or computer program can replace the human touch of a
doctor on his or her patient's

> The truth is, there is great hope for cancer right now.

life. Unfortunately, doctors'
abuse of technology is
another factor that has under-
mined the ability of the
physician to listen to and
observe the patient. While modernization saves doctors time and
effort, too often this saved time is allocated to the development
and use of more devices instead of giving more attention to the
patient, especially those with chronic diseases who need a lot of
our time. Consultation times become increasingly shorter as doctors continue to distance themselves from patients. The lure of
technology has alienated physicians from their true mission—
which is loving our patients, if not as much as we love ourselves,
certainly more than we love science and technology.

Is there a better way?

Following the money trail has shown us that in spite of real
medical advances, we are often blinded by the glitz and glitter of
a powerful medical machine from clearly following a path to a
permanent cure for cancer and other diseases. Although medical
research promises great things for the future and continually
dangles promises of cures before our eyes—they are always on
the horizon.

The truth is, there is great hope for cancer right now. We
must not limit our search for a cure to the parameters set for us
by this powerful medical machine. There is an exciting dimension of treatments and methods that have been proven successful and are continually working for patients right now,
sometimes in conjunction with more conventional treatments.
If you are willing to read on with an open mind, you are about to
discover some genuine alternatives that are gaining recognition
for their track record of facilitating cancer cures!

Section II

Considering Other Choices

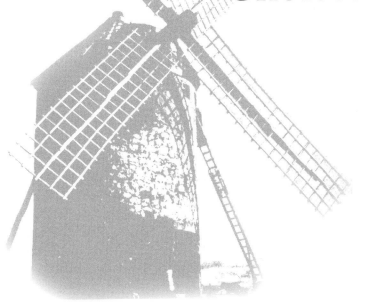

5 Exciting Cancer Treatments: Laetrile; Issels' Therapy

When I was twelve years old, because of an illness that kept me in bed for a few days, my mother gave me two enormous volumes to read to help me wile away the dreary hours. It was *The Adventures of Don Quixote* by Cervantes. When I first saw the size of the books, I decided I would only look at the illustrations. But soon I became so fascinated with the illustration that I found myself consumed in the story.

Although as a kid I enjoyed reading, *The Adventures of Don Quixote* was the first book to ever completely consume my imagination. It took away my desire for sleep; I devoured its pages night and day until I had finished the last page of both volumes.

The author, Cervantes, ingeniously portrayed the story of this madman—Don Quixote—who had incredible vision and passion powerful enough to change the world. The challenging concepts I read there about dreaming the impossible, fighting the unbeatable and reaching the unreachable had a profound influence on my young mind. They helped to shape and focus, perhaps even release, the destiny for my life that has propelled me to this moment. Even my closest friends criticize me for being an unredeemable dreamer and optimist in the face of fulfilling that destiny.

It was much later in my life before I realized I was living under the same roof with another true "Don Quixote." Even down to the lack of hair and lanky-build, my father resembled that good gentleman, and like Don Quixote, he was considered just another lunatic by most of his friends and colleagues. The truth was, as with Quixote, my father was simply a man captivated by the "madness" of an unreachable goal—the ultimate triumph over the hopelessness of those who are sick.

Treating the Whole Person

Ernesto Contreras, M.D., a celebrated cancer surgeon, armed himself with "quixotesque" or antiquated and bygone weaponry in the true practice of medicine. Today's cold professional has forgotten his time-tested art of healing, replacing it with the use of the latest technological advance. My father began to focus more on the patient than on the patient's tissue samples.

He fought valiantly all of his life for the triumph of good, justice, beauty and the love he had for medicine and for his patients. These are values many doctors have lost in the exercise of their profession. Too often they have been tossed aside in favor of fame, fortune and scientific development.

In the 1960s, my father was well known as one of the most promising doctors to graduate from the Army Medical in Mexico in the field of oncology. He did his residency in the Children's Hospital in Boston, Massachusetts, which is a Harvard hospital. However, in 1966 his life changed radically after taking a trip around the world with my mother, my oldest sister and her husband. As he explains in his autobiography, *To You, My Beloved Patient*, they visited Pergamum, an ancient Greek city of northwest Asia Minor in Mysia (now Turkey), where a group of scholars established a school of grammatical study in opposition to the scholars of the Alexandrian library.

A tour guide, knowing that my father was a doctor, decided to take him on an extended tour of the ruins of the ancient city. He showed my father an ancient sanitarium that was very different from the hospitals we now know. Patients had to pass through three different buildings to receive treatment. In the first building, patients met with religious counselors. They believed in the need of patients to be evaluated spiritually. In the second building, patients met with a psychologist of sorts who evaluated their mental well-being. Finally, in the third building, they received a physical evaluation. This approach to the practice of medicine shook my father. This ancient hospital in Pergamum was structured as a place for healing the whole man—body, mind and spirit. My father felt he had been enlightened by his visit to Pergamum; it was a light he had to follow.

Caring for our patients in the *totality* of their person is the goal of metabolic therapy.

Before taking this life-changing trip, my father had practiced the "exact" science of medicine, making diagnoses with the help of the microscope. After his voyage, he felt a tremendous burden that his work sentenced to death patients whom he didn't even know as the persons they were. Even worse, he had to explain to them that the treatments available to them promised suffering, not healing.

My father was convinced that modern medicine needed to adopt an approach more like the ancient one he had discovered in Pergamum that brought healing to the entire individual—body, mind and spirit. When he first began his alternative approach to medicine, my father called his method "holistic therapy." He recognized that to obtain the best results a doctor needed to treat the patient as a whole person—in the physical, emotional and spiritual attributes.

Since then the term *holistic* has been adopted by followers of many different philosophies, among them New Age therapists and others who have an anti-Christian religious philosophy, so we choose to refer to our approach as *metabolic therapy*. Metabolism involves the total function of our body that, to be carried out efficiently, must work in harmony in all its dimensions: body, mind and spirit. Caring for our patients in the *totality* of their person is the goal of metabolic therapy.

This goal is achieved through various alternative treatments including detoxification, diet, immune stimulation and antitumor agents. The objective of each treatment is to provide resources to create the best environment within our organism to fight disease, while at the same time making the cancer cells unwelcome.

My father's courage

My father didn't keep this viable approach to medicine to himself, but he began to divulge it to his colleagues in the medical community. He wanted to discuss the idea of loving the patient, taking into account spiritual and emotional needs as well as desperate physical conditions, especially in regard to cancer. As early as 1967, he reminded his colleagues of the atrocities effected by surgery, radiation and chemotherapy, and encouraged them to seek less aggressive, more natural and less toxic therapies for cancer treatment.

The response of my father's peers in the medical community to his "old-fashioned" approach was immediate. Applause? No, he was promptly expelled from the medical establishment and professionally exiled. Their judgment—the man had gone mad. But those taunts and humiliations along the way did not stop him in his quest to reach the unreachable star—a true cure for cancer.

My father's exile from the medical establishment was the blow exactly prescribed for him by the Divine Physician—God Himself. Though the enemies he faced were true giants—not only the incurable disease of cancer itself, but also his lack of acceptance in the medical establishment—he did not throw his hands up in despair. Like Don Quixote, he said, "I am going to engage them in fierce and unequal battle." He had encountered his divine destiny.

In the face of the harsh criticism of his colleagues, my father began to carry out what he considered to be his divine mission. Already excommunicated from the medical guild, he founded his own hospital, *The Oasis of Hope* (of which I am now director), and became a pioneer in the practice of holistic medicine and alternative therapies. There he practiced and promoted the idea that orthodox therapies, while useful in some aspects, should be applied in a less aggressive form along with alternative methods of healing.

Understanding cancer to be a systemic disease, he preached that proper diet and detoxification of the body were equal or superior to any therapeutic method, alternative or orthodox. He believed that rebuilding the immune system and strengthening the general health of the patient are important goals to pursuing healing. And he instituted programs to help patients with their emotional and spiritual challenges. He studied the causes of stress and sought for ways to enrich the spirit of his patients. As a result of my father's innovative approaches to his patients, the success of the hospital he founded to initiate these healing cancer therapies has a higher success rate today in the treatment of cancer than that of the famous oncological centers around the world.

When some scientists from the medical establishment have "evaluated" our treatment methods, they attempt to minimize our success by insinuating that our patients were misdiagnosed—that they didn't even have cancer. Or they assert that it is not the treatment we offer that helps the patient; rather, the patient merely experienced "spontaneous remission." To follow this logic, the sheer numbers of patients who have suddenly "gone into spontaneous remission," according to these scientists, would win for my father the recognition of being "the physician with most patients who experienced spontaneous remission in the history of medicine."

I deeply admire my father for his intelligence, knowledge and enormous clinical ability, as well as his human "touch" with patients. Their own testimonies reveal that after spending only a few minutes with Dr. Contreras they felt relief. But what I will always admire even more is his courage to make whatever sacrifice was necessary so that his patients could have access to healing "alternatives," in light of the fact that "accepted" treatments were so clearly ineffective. He was not intimidated when he lost his position in the medical community as a renowned scientist or when he was challenged by establishment oncologists or when authorities closed him down or when money was scarce. He didn't even shrink from the worst they could throw at him— that his prestige be tainted by their taunts of "quackery."

He faced this unbelievable persecution, always harboring in his heart the "call" to attend the suffering. For the love of his patients he bore all things, believed all things, hoped all things and endured all things. Thanks to unfaltering courage and his tireless efforts, less aggressive and more natural treatments are available to many cancer patients today.

A Legacy of Change

Much has changed since 1967 when my father challenged the windmills of the orthodox medical establishment with a wooden sword made from little more than the purity of his heart and a deep compassion for suffering patients. Today, more and more clinics, hospitals and private physicians embrace my father's holistic concepts of healing, once so firmly ridiculed.

According to Dr. Bruckheim of Tribune Media Services, a survey pointed out that 30 percent of all doctors frequently steer their patients to alternative therapies, 74 percent admit to having used unconventional remedies in their consultation rooms and 67 percent have occasionally sought the help of alternative doctors for their patients. Of those brave souls who have personally experimented with unorthodox methods, 91 percent say they would do so again.

One example is the M. D. Anderson Hospital, where they now practice conservative surgery for breast cancer. When my father promoted this kind of surgery thirty years ago he was called a quack. And the Mayo Clinic recently published a book on the power of nutrition, though thirty years ago my father was ridiculed for affirming that diet played an important role in the prevention and treatment of cancer. First they ridiculed his hypotheses; then they fought them "scientifically." Now they are using them to treat their patients.

Searching for a better way

Increasingly, the paradigm of thinking behind traditional medicine is shifting. The costly pursuit of a magic bullet to stop cancer has continued to elude us. That's partly because the processes within the body that break down and develop cancers are so complex and varied. There are too many genes to explore to advance the genetic approach to the disease in a timely way. And if people get hurt by new experimental therapies, drug makers may face thorny ethical and liability issues. The industry itself admits that there's a lot of hype, and investors may lose interest before scientists understand enough to bring effective products to market.

In addition, there is growing disillusion with traditional cancer therapies such as chemotherapy, radiation and radical surgeries, as we have discussed, which not only remove a tumor and a surrounding ring of affected tissue but also cut away large areas of healthy tissue and assault the body. Designed to attack the cancer tumor, these invasive treatments act instead like carpet bombs, destroying the valuable systems in your body that God created to help it fight disease and heal the body.

In a sense, the lack of a magic bullet to cure cancer is helping us in our pursuit of the coming cure for cancer. It is causing us to search for a better way and making us deal with hard questions and evaluate realistic expectations regarding the disease, the cure and our prospects for health.

Realistic expectations

What are your expectations? That is a question that I like all my patients to ponder when they come to the Oasis of Hope Hospital, because satisfaction and ultimate happiness depend on whether or not your expectations are met. And I want, as much as possible, a group of happy campers in my hospital.

The Coming Cancer Cure is an enticing title for this book; it creates specific expectations in the reader, which is precisely what I intend to do. But if I do not satisfy you, the reader, with real information that fulfills the expectations created by the title, I have failed, and you will be unhappy.

In this same way, oncologists in the present medical culture, along with researchers, pharmaceutical entrepreneurs and politicians, have created an expectation in the public for a cancer "cure." And because research, humanity's foremost hope in the war against cancer, has come short of this expectation in spite of so many years of work and so much money invested, everyone is unhappy.

Expectations must be realistic, or they will become defeating. Unrealistic expectations are the surest way to unhappiness; they will lead you on a wild goose chase to one failure after frustrating failure. Imagine that in order for my wife to be happy she expects me to grow five inches taller. She would be in trouble! I cannot meet her expectations, so she is doomed to unhappiness. But if she asked that I lose ten pounds so that I would look better and live longer, that is a realistic expectation that I could, and should, fulfill to make her happy.

My desire is to help you build your own down-to-earth expectations for your possibilities for health, not the unrealistic ones that doctors, the media or the market has planted in your minds. To that end I will present a variety of *alternative* treatments for cancer that will open doors for everyone to consider, whether you need to prevent, destroy or control the disease. These are realistic methods that will help you achieve happiness and be victorious over this dreaded terrorist.

As beauty is in the eye of the beholder, so victory is in the heart of the fighter. Usually what separates the champion from the rest of the competitors is his or her emotional fortitude. A fighter that believes he has no chance of winning is easily defeated. No matter how strong the body may be, if the mind is weak failure is imminent. But when the mind is strong, no matter how weak the body, the competitor will always have a fighting chance. It was one of my father's patients who christened my father's work *The Oasis of Hope*. Doctors sent her home to die, filled with a sense of hopelessness. When she visited my father, he restored her hope, helping her realize that she still had her heart with which she could fight. And she rose victorious to the challenge.

The aim of our therapies at Oasis of Hope Hospital is not to destroy tumors. Yes, you read it right; getting rid of a tumor is not our primary goal. Why? Because, in general, this is an unrealistic expectation. Consider how many decades of failures represented by so many lives lost that this attitude of oncologists and patients—this no-matter-what-it-takes-just-get-rid-of-the-tumor attitude—has achieved.

For the real cause of cancer, scientific evidence points an accusing finger toward the inability of the immune system to resist external and internal aggressions against the body. These assaults finally break down the defenses of people's bodies, unfortunately in growing numbers, resulting in their developing a form of cancer.

It is the inability of the body to resist these assaults that I consider my primary enemy rather than tumors. Building the body's defenses against disease is the priority of metabolic therapies. This is the paradigm shift oncology needs to acknowledge in order to improve its negative record in the treatment of cancer.

Though cancer has proven itself to be a formidable foe, we still must answer the question of why 40 to 50 percent of us develop cancer and the others do not, when all of us are exposed to the same external and internal aggressions. Obviously the "lucky" ones have innate resources that keep their immune systems honest.

I work very hard at the Oasis of Hope Hospital to provide the necessary resources (physical, emotional and spiritual) to my patients for them to heal themselves. In some cases, they will achieve a "spontaneous remission," but this is not the only means of success available. As I mentioned before, many of our patients die of "old age" with cancer, not because of it. If you cannot get rid of it, the next best solution is to make it your partner. Instead of fighting it (literally) to the death with aggressive treatments alone, aid yourself with natural resources to fight it from within.

When your body's offensive mechanisms are in top shape, they have the potential to neutralize cancer's life-threatening growth and keep its destructive potential at bay. These offensive mechanisms can create a peaceable arrangement sort of like a good ol' marriage: "You don't bother me, and I don't bother you." And there you have it, a more realistic expectation.

What I am proposing is not just a medical paradigm shift; I want to change the entire medical approach to the treatment of attacking disease at its roots. The Hippocratic philosophy of "do no harm" is just not enough; we must advance into the Christian model of "loving our neighbor as we love ourselves." This is a principle that is too often ignored by doctors when they offer scientifically justified treatments to patients that they would not submit to themselves.

> **Cancer victims can become cancer victors who consider the possibility for survival.**

The promising research for the development of a cure for cancer is exciting. I pray that medical cure will be available for my children so they can grow up without this terrible threat. In the meantime, cancer victims can become cancer victors who consider the possibility for survival. Too often cancer victims feel doomed with the "cancer equals death" paradigm. At Oasis of

Hope, we have changed that paradigm to "resources equal life"; that is a realistic expectation that opens the doors wide for cancer victims to become cancer victors.

Spontaneous Remissions

One of the most wonderful successes of the metabolic therapy approach is that it unlocks the innate healing power of the body. Believe it or not, your body is able to fight cancer on its own, even in the final stages. Many oncologists witness what we call "spontaneous remissions" even in those with cancer in the final stages. This occurs because the body has learned how to stop the cancer all by itself. It is a fascinating metabolic feat that traditional cancer researchers have overlooked. But it's a cornerstone for alternative therapies that support your body's own powerful healing mechanisms, helping your body bring cancer into submission.

Rather than carpet-bombing your body with highly toxic chemicals and burning it with destructive radiation that tears down your body's own cancer-fighting systems, alternative therapies trust the body's ability to fight disease and attempt to support it intelligently in this effort.

All of our bodies have cancer cells in them. The difference is that some of our bodies are effectively removing those cancer cells and maintaining a balanced state of good health while those who develop cancer do not. Alternative therapies attempt to build up the body's own resources, while at the same time fighting the cancer in the most noninvasive, nondestructive ways possible for each individual patient.

In our hospital we involve the patient in the treatment as well as the decision-making process. We never use therapies that deteriorate the quality of life. Instead, we provide patients with treatments that improve the quality of their lives. Sometimes we use an orthodox treatment if it's necessary and we know it will improve the patient's health. For example, if a patient's tumor is blocking the digestive tract, natural therapies would be inadequate because they take a long time to reduce tumor size. The patient's life is obviously threatened by the blockage in a matter of hours or days. In this case, surgery not only improves the quality of life for the patient, but it also saves his life.

In the same way, there are situations in which chemotherapy and radiation may be helpful. Even though we know that tumor reduction is not permanent with these therapies, it could give us the time needed for the alternative therapy to work effectively. We prefer chemotherapy treatments that are administered directly into a tumor through a catheter, rather than subject a cancer patient's entire body to dangerously toxic chemicals. Never would we administer chemotherapy and radiation at standard, and oftentimes lethal, dosages when we know that the risks far outweigh the benefits, putting not only the patient's well-being at stake, but also his or her very life.

Patients need a treatment that will attack the root of the problem. Natural therapies destroy tumors slowly through internal offensive mechanisms. These nontoxic therapies give the body the weapons it needs to fight illness. They do not attack the symptoms of cancer; they treat the foundation of the illness.

Laetrile—a Legacy of Hope

My father is the most famous pioneer in the use of Laetrile, which is also called amygdalin and vitamin B_{17}. He is the hero to those who have been healed, though he has been criticized by doctors who don't believe Laetrile has any therapeutic value. This naturally occurring antitumor agent has created much debate, but I have personally witnessed positive results with its use.

Chemically speaking, Laetrile is a diglucoside, which is a sugar with a cyanide radical. It exists in all seeds, except citrus, and in many plants. Egyptian doctors used it for curative purposes from the time of the pharaohs, and records show that Chinese herbalists used it in the year 2800 B.C. Laetrile is a successful, but greatly misunderstood cancer treatment.

The Hunza diet

Researchers became interested in Laetrile when it was learned that the Hunza tribes who live in the Himalayas enjoy one of the lowest cancer rates in the world.[1] The Hunzas are one of the few people groups in the world reputed to be especially long lived. The Hunzas also enjoy an unspoiled environment and eat a completely natural diet with a low caloric rate that helps to account for their unusual longevity.[2]

Of all of their organically grown food, perhaps their favorite and one of their dietary mainstays is the apricot—one of the best sources of amygdalin. Apricot orchards are everywhere in Hunza communities, and family economic status is measured by how many apricot trees they have under cultivation.[3]

They eat their apricots in season and dry a great deal more in the sun for eating throughout the long, cold winter. They purée dried apricots and mix them with snow to make ice cream. But that's not all. The Hunzas remove the seeds from the fruits, crack them and remove the almond-like nuts. The women hand-grind these kernels with stone mortars, then squeeze the meal between a hand stone and a flat rock to press the oil. The oil from these apricot kernels is used in cooking, as a salad dressing on fresh garden greens and even as a facial lotion.[4]

Pueblo Indians' recipe

The Pueblo Indians of Taos, New Mexico, traditionally eat many foods rich in amygdalin. Not coincidentally, cancer is rare among this people, too.[5] Robert G. Houston, who has written several articles on the Pueblos, was given the following recipe by the Indians while living among them to research a book on cancer prevention:

> In a glass of milk or juice, mix a tablespoon of honey with a quarter ounce (two dozen) freshly ground apricot kernels, or one kernel for every ten pounds of body weight.

Houston wrote that the drink was so delicious that he had it every day.[6]

Biochemist Dr. Ernest T. Krebs Jr. discovered that it was amygdalin that was protecting these people from developing cancer. Krebs called it vitamin B_{17},[7] inferring that a large supply would inhibit cancer from developing. The definition of *vitamin* is a substance that when insufficient causes disease, and when absent, death. In other words, it is absolutely necessary for good function and ultimately life. Amygdalin, although monumental, is not necessary for life and thus not a vitamin. Nevertheless the name of vitamin B_{17} stuck.

Already judged as therapeutically ineffective, health officials claimed that Laetrile was also a poison.[8] They ignored the fact that virtually every fruit contains some amounts of Laetrile. To date, we have treated more than forty thousand patients with high dosages of amygdalin, and we have never had one case of cyanide poisoning.

A success story

"The cures for all man's diseases already exist in the world around us. It is the task of science to recognize them," said Selman Abraham Waksman, a famous pharmacology expert.[9] Amygdalin is a natural chemotherapy, effective and completely nontoxic. Furthermore, when the amygdalin breaks down, it produces a very strong painkiller, another blessing for patients with tumors.

Amygdalin has been proven extraordinarily effective in the treatment of common tumors such as carcinomas of the prostate, breast, colon and lungs as well as lymphomas. Twenty years ago, German scientists reported that enzymes that break up proteins could aid amygdalin by synergism, or the energy released by combining them. Since then these enzymes have been given together with amygdalin, resulting in an improvement of our statistics.

Let me share with you the story of one of my father's patients.

My father has records of thousands of patients who enjoyed similar results. This man had a primary tumor in the kidney with metastasis in the lung and was told he had less than a year to live. He came to my father in 1987 to take Laetrile and receive metabolic therapy.

If I showed you the x-rays from 1987, and then showed you the follow-up x-rays taken in 1994 and 1999, you would see tumors in all of them. The patient still has tumors, but he has survived with a cancer for twelve years that should have killed him in less than twelve months. And he was feeling great and going strong the last time I talked with him.

Of course, Laetrile is not the only alternative therapy we offer at the Oasis of Hope Hospital, though we have been a leader in the use of Laetrile as a part of our cancer treatment program. We are committed to the exploration and use of many alternative therapies, as well as orthodox treatments for cancer when needed, as long as they prolong life and guard an individual's quality of life as well.

Dramatically Superior Results

Since 1963, one hundred thousand patients have been treated at the Oasis of Hope Hospital founded by Dr. Ernesto Contreras Sr. Patients have come here from every part of the world seeking cancer therapies and treatment approaches pioneered by the Contreras doctors, specifically the *Metabolic Therapy.*

In 1981 we conducted a retrospective study to document the five-year survival rates of our cancer patients. It is important to note that 95 percent of these patients came to us with stage IV cancers after conventional therapy had failed to help them. They had been sent home to die.

We treated them with our metabolic therapy, and the results were encouraging. Our overall five-year rate for all types of cancer was 30 percent. We also noted that 86 percent of our patients outlived their prognosis and reported an improvement in their quality of life.

Malignancies in the lung, breast, colon and prostate are the most prevalent in our experience. For this reason, we designed a prospective study on the efficacy of metabolic therapy focused on these advanced stage IV cancers. In the table below, we compare our results against those from clinical trials with conventional therapies.

Type of cancer (Distant*)	Number of patients	Five-year survival rate (%)	
		Oasis	Conventional**
Lung Cancer	200	30%	2%
Breast Cancer	130	39%	21%
Colon Cancer	150	30%	8%
Prostate Cancer	600	86%	33%

*   Distant: A malignant cancer that has spread to parts of the body remote from the primary tumor either by direct extension or by discontinuous metastasis to distant organs, tissues or via the lymphatic system to distant lymph nodes.

** Source: American Cancer Society, *Cancer Facts & Figures*, 2001

The Oasis statistics when compared to the conventional statistics are dramatically better. What makes these results astounding to me is the difference between the Oasis group and the conventional group. The Oasis patients had already undergone surgery, radiation or chemotherapy. They had endured the hair loss, nausea, burns and devastation of their energy levels and immune systems.

Those in the conventional group had no previous treatment to damage their general condition. They had a fresh start. We can only speculate on the better results we could achieve with patients who would avoid conventional therapy before they arrive at the Oasis of Hope.

In spite of the impressive results, our studies were rejected by all peer-reviewed medical journals. The only studies that these groups recognize are single-drug double-blind clinical trials. Our study just didn't meet those criteria. In fact, our results depend on a combination of therapies. This makes it difficult to single out one active agent, and this is the objective of cancer research. Scientists want to identify the means, and we have focused completely on the end result.

Our results in lung cancer were so dramatic, however, that one group of oncological authorities did invite us to make a presentation at the World Congress on Cancer in Buenos Aires. Unfortunately, the Congress coordinators canceled our participation at the last minute due to opposition from some outspoken doctors. Once again, those who insisted that the results were secondary and that our study did not adhere to their guidelines were able to silence us.

In the past, financial restraints and negativity from the oncological community have hindered us from conducting standard double-blind clinical trials. But the legal and medical environment is changing as more and more people demand access to alternative medicine. The governments in the United States and Mexico have already established offices of alternative medicine in their health departments. The Ministry of Health in Mexico has approved our application for a clinical research organization (CRO), and we are now positioning ourselves for research grants. We intend to conduct the necessary trials to publish the results in an effort to make valid therapies available to people in any part of the world.

We have never been on a crusade to prove the value of alternative therapies. In fact, we have often been criticized for our use of conventional medicine. We keep focused on our ultimate goal, the total well-being of our patients. We try not to limit our patients to either alternative or orthodox therapies. We offer them what are the most effective and least harmful options. Our approach complements conventional medicine with natural elements and mind/spirit support. To our critics who say that we do not utilize pure science, we would like to remind them: Medicine is much more than science; it is a healing art.[10]

Issels' Cancer Treatment

Josef M. Issels, M.D. is remembered worldwide as the foremost pioneer of the holistic integrative approach to cancer and chronic degenerative disease. Over 90 percent of all Dr. Issels' patients were suffering from progressive metastatic cancer. He developed a very comprehensive logistic treatment system, which he first published in 1953 and administered to approximately fifteen thousand cancer patients in the hospital and clinic he founded in 1951 at Lake Tegernsee near Munich, Germany.

Research has shown that every vertebrate organism is constantly threatened by cancer cells whose formation is a daily occurrence. Not every newly produced cancer cell leads to a tumor, as the body possesses a natural defense system.

Dr. Issels' conclusions from this experience in his holistic concept of the development of chronic degenerative disease and malignancy serve as the foundation for his comprehensive treatment strategy. This effective strategy attends to both the disease symptoms and the causes and preconditions for the development of these symptoms.

In the case of cancer, the treatment is not only directed at the malignant tumor, but also at the correction of the preconditions for the formation of the tumor. It aims at the restoration of the natural defense, repair and regulatory mechanisms of the cancer-afflicted person as a whole.

The Issels Treatment opens up the following therapeutic possibilities:

- Treatment of cancer of all types and stages offering a considerable chance of recovery even for patients in advanced stages who have exhausted all standard treatments

- Follow-up treatment to reduce the risk of recurrence after standard cancer therapies through restoration of the patient's defense and repair functions

- Nontoxic preventive treatment for patients at risk (genetic predisposition coupled with environmental challenges) and those with precancerous lesions

- Preparatory treatment prior to surgery, radiation and chemotherapy to reduce complications and in qualified cases, to render inoperable tumors operable

- Treatment of chronic diseases that are untreatable by standard methods

Minding the state of the body

It is not the purpose of immunotherapy to replace surgery, radiation and chemotherapy. These "localized" treatments have their place within the integrative approach to cancer. On their own, however, they cannot be expected to be the answer to a chronic systemic disorder, although they have given their utmost in removing its symptom, the tumor.

Following Issels' regimen, an enormous amount of treatment is provided to the patient to restore his or her body back to top immune function and to remove any outside factors, such as toxins, that contributed to the disease process. Restoring all organ, neural and detoxification systems and intestinal floral weaknesses is part of the total restoration of the body to its precancerous condition.

Issels' extensive restorative treatment used together with conventional cancer methods has been proven to increase the survivor's rate from 50 percent to 87 percent and lower the recurrence rate from 50 percent to 13 percent. Issels' treatment has also been shown to raise the rate of spontaneous remission from 2 percent to 17 percent in cases of incurable cancers. This rate of complete long-term remissions is considered remarkable within the medical community. (For a technical discussion of

Issels' Therapy, please see Appendix H.)

Walking With a "Don Quixote"

Breakthroughs in alternative therapies have only begun to receive some of the recognition they deserve. And those who went on a quest, laying down their lives, their reputations and their fortunes to fight the giant windmills of cancer, are discovering that their gallant efforts were worth it. More and more lives are being saved every day. And as mainstream research is being forced to see what these brave Don Quixotes were able to see so many years ago, there is great hope that the combined efforts of all sides of the research spectrum will finally slay this cruel terrorist.

The greatest privilege God has given me is to walk shoulder to shoulder as the son and disciple of a "Don Quixote" and grasp the ideal practice of medicine—that it is truly an art-science, filled with love and hope for patients. My father's passionate, loving "madness" empowered him to reach for incredible victories that even his peers in the medical community thought were unreachable.

And it enabled me to discover my destiny to continue his brave struggle to bring to suffering humanity the coming cancer cure. As we continue intensive research, demanding cancer to reveal the secrets of its destructive power, we learned much from earlier pioneers and our studies as well, and we experienced a wonderful breakthrough into yet another effective cancer cure—Ozone Therapy.

6 Ozone Therapy: A Potential Cure

F ernando Bonetti (not his real name) was dying. His skin, the white of his eyes and his mucus were tainted yellow. I knew that all of his internal organs, including his brain, were invaded with a toxic waste material called bilirubin, which is secreted by the liver.

Under normal conditions, bilirubin is excreted by the bile and is a bitter, alkaline, brownish-yellow or greenish-yellow fluid that is stored in the gallbladder. It is then discharged into the duodenum where it aids in the emulsification, digestion and absorption of fats.

In Fernando's case, his liver was so damaged that it was unable to get rid of this toxic fluid, and the bilirubin started accumulating in all of his tissues, causing all kinds of symptoms ranging from itching to brain malfunction. Fernando's bilirubin levels were about thirty times above normal. Because of his liver failure, his body was wasting away. He looked like a jaundiced concentration camp survivor.

His prognosis was actually worse than his worst fears. He knew he was deathly ill, but he clung to the hope of recovery. After viewing his films, however, and finding innumerable malignant tumors that had invaded his liver and then reviewing his pathologist's report of a hepatoma, one of the most deadly malignancies, I was not sure there was much we could do for him. Nevertheless, Fernando's faith sustained me, and we began to develop a therapeutic approach to combat the physical deficiencies provoked by the liver cancer.

Fernando was the ideal patient. He was always smiling despite his torturous pain, always adding hopeful comments, always on time for the treatments. He was truly upbeat in the face of malaise caused by the liver insufficiency and the fatigue resulting from malnutrition caused by constant nausea and abdominal distention.

He came to me looking for alternatives. He had received all of the treatments modern oncology had to offer, but they failed him; he had been sent home to die—a sentence he could not face as a young man at the age of thirty-eight.

Many people think of alternative therapy in terms of herbs, diet and prayer. It involves much more than these elements, though they are a vital part of alternative therapy. Fernando's aggressive, fast-growing tumor needed to be stopped in its tracks, and quickly. Otherwise his few remaining functioning liver cells were going to succumb to the invasion of the malignant ones, which would result in certain death.

His liver insufficiency was a big obstacle. All medicines are metabolized in the liver, which was incapacitated as we have described. With any medication we gave him we risked precipitating the end of his liver function, and thereby killing him. Therefore, we decided to treat him with oxygen, the only element that would not interfere with his failing liver.

Oxygen? you may ask.

Yes, oxygen!

Before you dismiss this whole idea as a hoax, let me continue Fernando's incredible story. Fernando did not die as statistically and medically expected. Instead, as we treated him he began to improve from all of his symptoms, and after three short months of therapeutic intervention, he was completely well. Not only was he feeling good, a CT of his liver demonstrated the absence of any tumors. Fernando had a new liver!

The Theory of Oxygen Therapy

In 1998, our Clinical Research Organization (CRO) at Oasis of Hope Hospital developed a research protocol using blood oxygenation and ozonation as an antitumor therapy. The idea was not new. In fact, German scientists have been using ozone, a kind of very reactive superoxygen (three atoms of oxygen-O_3), in the treatment of cancer and other diseases for several decades based on the discovery of Otto Warburg, who won a Nobel Prize in 1931 for the discovery.

Warburg discovered that all normal body cells are *obligate aerobes* (they need oxygen), whereas all cancer cells are *partial anaerobes* (they don't like oxygen). In other words, cancer cells prefer to grow in an oxygen-poor environment. Based on that evidence, it was believed that by sending oxygen to cancer cells, which dreaded its presence, they would be destroyed.[1]

Since the 1960s when these facts were published, many scientists have tried—albeit unsuccessfully—to use oxygen to combat cancer. Ozone, a form of compressed oxygen, has been researched specifically for this purpose by many scientists. Other methods such as intravenous peroxide and pure oxygen breathing have produced disappointing results.[2]

Like so many great thinkers, Warburg was far ahead of his time even in predicting what was necessary to successfully use oxygen in cancer therapy. He had concluded that the only way to combat cancer with oxygen was by increasing blood oxygen transportation to such an extent that the venous blood would contain sufficient oxygen to saturate with oxygen all growing body cells.

Unfortunately, the oxygen level in the veins is normally very low. While most of the circulating blood in our bodies, about 70 percent, is running through our veins, it is normally oxygen-poor, toxin-rich blood. Arterial blood, which is rich in oxygen, makes up only 17 percent of the body's total blood volume. (The other 13 percent of blood is inside the organs.) That means that most of the blood running through our body does not contain very much oxygen. The technology needed to apply Warburg's theory, getting life-giving oxygen into the veins where it could destroy cancer cells, was only achieved decades after Warburg discovered its potential benefit. And when first discovered, the technology was not applied to cancer therapy.

Therapeutic Ozone

For many years, we at the Oasis of Hope Hospital have researched all methods of hyper-oxygenation in the hope of helping our patients. But the problem to using this therapy successfully lies in what Warburg suspected: that healing results could not be achieved unless there was a sufficient amount of oxygen in all of the venous blood (the veins).

The first breakthrough for using oxygen to combat cancer came with the discovery of therapeutic ozone, which makes it possible for blood to be oxygenated when exposed to ozone. In fact, this gas can be directly injected into a patient's vein. This form of gas immediately disassociates in the blood into oxygen, which is absorbed by the hemoglobin, and peroxide into the plasma, so no air embolisms are created.

Whereas quickly injecting a person with a few cc's (cubic centimeters) of intravenous air can kill him or her, it is possible to safely inject ozone very slowly—from 80 to 100 cc's—with positive results. But even this method does not increase the amount of oxygen in the blood very much, at most an insignificant 10 percent, and its effects last only for a few minutes.

Through years of research at the Oasis of Hope Hospital, we have been able to successfully establish oxygen therapy that makes good use of Warburg's discoveries. Our therapy not only significantly increases the oxygen levels in venous blood, but it also promotes the synthesis of oxygen inside malignant cells. We call our therapy TMO, which stands for *Terapia Metabolica Oasis*. It is this therapy that helped Fernando recover from his desperate condition.

A second wonderful breakthrough came with the development of therapeutic ozone. This new ozone did not disassociate so quickly, which allows the increased oxygen level of the blood to last longer. The important thing with this therapy is to dramatically increase the oxygen supply in the veins, which can only happen when the blood is exposed to therapeutic ozone for longer periods of time.

Though ozone can damage the lungs when it is inhaled, other human cells are not damaged by it at all. Bypassing the lungs was not complicated because ozone can be directly injected into a patient's vein. As mentioned earlier, this form of gas immediately disassociates in the blood into oxygen, which is absorbed by the hemoglobin, and peroxide into the plasma so no air embolisms are created. This disassociation of ozone in blood into its components is a one, two punch against disease. Oxygen enriches all tissues, and peroxide triggers a cascade of beneficial immune-stimulating mechanisms that are especially devastating to malignant cells.

I found other scientists in Italy, England and Africa who were using total blood ozonation through an extra-corporeal loop, a method developed for dialysis in the treatment of kidney failure. In dialysis a filter is perfused with chemical agents that remove the toxins from the blood that the failed kidneys are not excreting. For the purpose of oxygenating the blood, ozone is perfused through the filter. This innovative application of a proven method (dialysis) has given us the possibility of circulating and exposing all of the patient's blood to ozone for a prolonged period of time, about sixty minutes. During ozonation the typically oxygen-poor venous blood is hyper-oxygenated to about 750 percent.

The Italians have discovered that the disassociation of ozone not only increases delivery of oxygen to tissues, but it also generates the production of what we call Reactive Oxygen Species (ROS). One of these species is the well-known hydrogen peroxide. Hydrogen peroxide, a free radical, paradoxically benefits the cellular environment due to a potent antioxidation stimulus that, in the long run, eventually helps cells to resist oxidative stress.

The other ROS are called ozonides and lipid hydroperoxides. They trigger potent immune-stimulating, antitumor biochemical mechanisms that induce the production of cytokines, interleukins, interferon, tumor necrosis factor (TNF) and alpha and beta transforming growth factors. These potent immune factors contribute in the destruction of malignant cells or at least in creating an adverse environment to the tumor, making it more liable for other cancer-killing agents.[3]

In order to use large amounts of ozone without the danger of causing a gaseous embolism, we utilized an extra-corporeal loop similar to the kind of loop used in blood dialysis. With this device, we could hyper-oxygenate the blood for hours at a time. Not only does this method keep cancer tumors from growing any larger than they already are, but we've found that cancer tumors also shrink—some even die—after only a few sessions of the extra-corporeal blood ozone exposure. The best part of all is that there are no negative side effects![4]

Destroying cancer cells is extremely important and is the worthy goal of conventional cancer treatments. Surgery, radiation and chemotherapy do destroy cancer cells. But, statistically, though these conventional treatments achieve the goal of destroying tumors, that does not necessarily translate to the survival of the patient. For that reason, using nontoxic, nonaggressive methods of tumor destruction such as oxygen therapy are far more desirable than methods that are so toxic they often kill the patient.

Encouraging results

This therapy was a "magic bullet" for Fernando. I wish I could tell you that all of the patients that undergo ozone therapy have the same miraculous results as Fernando; I cannot. Nevertheless, the preliminary results of ozone therapy for the treatment of cancer are extremely encouraging.

In four out of ten patients, ozone therapy has been able to stop tumor growth or reduce tumor size from between 10 to 30 percent in a very short period of time (twelve treatments in twenty-one days). And this noninvasive treatment is without side effects for the patient. In all prospective clinical trials, there are patient characteristics, status of the disease and other factors that will determine whether or not an individual can be included in this therapy. Fernando actually did not fit into our criteria. Therefore, we adjusted his treatment according to his very particular needs. Those adjustments probably saved his life.

As effective as oxygen can be to shrink and destroy tumors, we understand that destroying the tumor only represents half the battle. Tumor destruction will not diminish the recurrent threat of cancer unless the ultimate cause is addressed: the metabolic failure of the immune system. After all, cancer is, as we now know, a systemic disease.

Attacking Cancer at the Roots

As I have stated, the aim of the therapy programs at the Oasis of Hope Hospital is to attack the roots of cancer, addressing all the factors that break down the body's defenses and allow disease to attack it. Both external and internal immune-suppressing factors are taken into account when treating a patient. We are determined to help restore the power of the body, mind and spirit to be able to maintain health as God ordained it to do.

Our programs address the problems of the patient's entire system, beginning with the elimination of built-up toxins in the body through a comprehensive detoxification program. We also build the body's defenses through nutrition and supplementation and by removing all cancer-causing substances from the diet. These simple but vital measures give the body an important boost toward rebuilding the immune system to its God-ordained power and vigor. Vitamins, minerals, enzymes and phytochemicals all strengthen the body's ability to fight against disease.

In addition, often some of the greatest factors robbing the

immune system do not come from the body at all. Destructive emotional and spiritual factors take a greater toll upon an individual's body than most of us realize. At Oasis of Hope, we have created an atmosphere where patients can participate in activities that will help them resolve the effects of destructive emotions.

Patients learn to reduce stress through music and prayer; they take part in group therapy and receive personal support. For those who wish to participate in these activities, they will find them to be an opportunity to establish or strengthen a personal relationship with God. We have found that treating the whole person affected by a life-threatening disease brings much greater results of healing than simply attacking a symptom, such as a tumor.

We continually confront the myth that cancer is a tumor and attempt to change that treatment paradigm for the reality of treating cancer as the systemic disease that it is. Learning to cope with a systemic disease requires a patient to focus on many different areas of need in order to realize the healing they seek. Certain lifestyle changes are required if a patient expects to restore the body from its broken, diseased state to a healthy one. Diet is one of the important areas that must be considered, since what we eat has a great effect on our immune systems and our health.

7 Gerson's Empirical Evidence for Diet Therapy

Max Gerson, M.D. was born in Wongrowitz, Germany in 1881. His personal experiences as a migraine sufferer led him to begin researching the potential of diet as a cure for his ills. During his research, Dr. Gerson discovered that not only did his migraines improve, but while following his "migraine diet," his skin tuberculosis was cured as well.

The famous Nobel Prize winner Dr. Schweitzer and his wife became close friends with Gerson after his diet cured Mrs. Schweitzer of lung tuberculosis when all other methods had failed. Schweitzer's own Type II diabetes was also cured by Gerson's nutritional method. Gerson then went on to study how other diseases would respond to treatment through nutritional methods.[1]

In 1924 Gerson was invited by noted thoracic surgeon Ferdinand Sauerbruch to test his dietary treatment in a special lupus clinic under the support of the Bavarian government at the University of Munich. Sauerbruch recounts that 446 patients of 450 recovered.[2] Later his dietary method extended to pulmonary tuberculosis as well. The Gerson-Sauerbruch-Hermannsdorfer diet was widely used in Germany and became the subject of Gerson's first book in 1934.[3]

During the late twenties and early thirties Gerson had several experiences that educated him regarding diet and degenerative disease. As a member of the State Board of Health, appointed by the Prussian government, he was given extraordinary laboratory support for a clinical trial of diet in pulmonary tuberculosis.[4] Here Gerson was able to track minute fluctuations in the patient's mineral metabolism and also in the chemical composition of the foods he prescribed.

In 1928, a woman who had jaundice and a hopeless case of liver cancer insisted that he give her a diet for cancer. Reluctantly, he wrote her a diet after he obtained a written agreement that she would not hold him responsible for the outcome. Having taken up this challenge against his will, with no hope of success, Gerson was astounded when his patient seemed fully recovered in six months.[5] In quick succession, he had the same good results with two patients with inoperable stomach cancer.[6]

In 1935–1936, Gerson moved to Paris where he continued his work with good results in three of seven cancer patients.[7]

Gradually, out of his experience and his reading, Dr. Gerson formed a unitary theory of degenerative disease that included cancer. The theory rested on one of the oldest and most pervasive concepts in the history of medicine—the healing power of nature.[8]

Diligently pursuing the latest research results in physiology, biochemistry and immunology, Gerson integrated this research into an understanding of healing called "the physician within," or the natural powers of resistance. Today we call it the *immune system*.

The Gerson Therapy

In his last book, which is the classic volume of the Gerson Therapy, Dr. Gerson gives his insightful understanding of the origins of cancer:

In my opinion, cancer is not a problem of deficiencies of hormones, vitamins and enzymes. It is not a problem of allergies or infections, viral or others; it is not a poisoning through some metabolic or external substance (carcinogen), nor caused by a genetic factor. It is an accumulation of numerous damaging factors, in combination causing the deterioration of the entire metabolism when the liver has been progressively impaired.

In other words, it is a mistake to search for THE cause of cancer; there is no single cause of the disease. With metabolic healing by the Gerson Therapy, it has been our experience that even presumably genetic cancers can be cured. The genes may well predispose the person to a weakness of the liver and/or the immune system; the damage is reversible![9]

To prove this point, Gerson published his *Results of 50 Cases,* all of which arrived in terminal condition to begin his treatment. Many of those published "patients" who were young at that time are living now, having survived forty-five years, and are in their seventies and eighties. Over the course of sixty years, the Gerson Therapy has amply demonstrated its enormous potential and power to heal, curing many patients classified as "incurable" in terms of conventional medicine.

One more recent patient, a professor of medicine at the Fukushima College of Medicine (a medical school in northern Japan), discovered that he had developed colon cancer. When the problem was diagnosed in 1992, he submitted to surgery to remove the tumor. In the course of the surgery, visual inspection and a subsequent biopsy also revealed metastases to his liver. He refused chemotherapy and, instead, followed the Gerson Therapy, along with some additional immune therapy. He recovered completely and remains well as of December 2001. He also prescribed the Gerson Therapy for twelve additional cancer patients. He describes his experience in the book he wrote in 1998 on the Gerson Therapy (available in Japanese only; not translated into English).

Gerson understood that cancer changes the body's normal sodium/potassium balance, which is already impacted by modern diet. Therefore, he used foods low in sodium (no salt), high in potassium and rich in vitamins A, C and oxidizing enzymes in his nutritional method.

For the first four to six weeks, his patients were forbidden to eat fats and dairy products. But above all, Gerson blamed sodium for altering molecular chemistry and opening the door to cancerous growths.[10]

What he suspected has now been proven. Colon cancer is often accompanied by an environment of very low potassium, and other cancers are also attended by alterations in electrical and mineral states.[11]

Researcher G. N. Ling and his associates showed that damaged cells partially return to their normal state in high potassium/low sodium environments, which explained the remarkable tissue repair that Gerson sometimes saw in his formerly debilitated patients.[12]

Gerson's cancer patients were given hourly glasses of freshly prepared vegetable and fruit juices to supply enzymes and potassium-rich minerals. He also had his patients drink two to three glasses of the juice of calves' liver pressed with carrots. In addition to vitamin A, the liver juice supplied iron and copper, which have been shown to impact immunity.[13]

Although the American Medical Association at the time dismissed the idea that diet played an important role in curing cancer, recent researchers have proven Gerson's theories to be correct. (To review specific aspects of this research, please turn to Appendix E.)

The immune system—your body's healing power

Gerson believed that the inflammation that occurs is a visible manifestation that the body is healing itself. He believed that every defense and healing power of the body depends on the capacity of the body to produce what he called an "allergic inflammation."

In his studies on cancer, he noted that fluid from a normal inflammation metabolism kills cancer cells, but blood serum does not. German researcher G. von Bergmann concluded from this that cancer occurs when the body can no longer produce this healing inflammatory reaction.[14]

Gerson took this one step farther, surmising that a physician could help restore the vital power of inflammation, even in patients with advanced stages of cancer who lacked this immune response. He concluded if cancer was a degenerative disease caused by the cumulative effect of inadequate nutrition with foods grown in soils depleted by artificial fertilizers and poisoned by toxic insecticides and herbicides, doctors must respond by replenishing the cancer patient's body.[15]

To Gerson, surgery, chemotherapy and radiation represented a superficial, symptomatic treatment, for the real problems lay in a poisoned metabolism.[16]

On guard against toxins and deficiencies

Dr. Gerson emphasized that a normal, healthy body has a strong ability to heal (i.e., infections, colds, flu or injuries). This natural ability, when lost through dangerous lifestyles, has to be restored if the body is to be helped to heal. With the proper nutrients and elimination of toxins, this can be done. In other words, with intensive detoxification and flooding the organism with fresh, living, organic nutrients, the body recovers.

According to Gerson, many factors depress the body's defenses and contribute to the onset of a malignancy. Above all, toxicity and deficiency of our environment hold the keys to causing disease.

First, toxicity in the air, water and soil; processed foods; over-the-counter, prescription and "recreational" drugs; household chemicals; industrial and occupational toxins—these all overwhelm the body's immune system and allow the start of disease.

For example, a seemingly innocent "necessary" to our daily lives that contributes especially to breast and lymphatic cancers is the use of deodorants and/or antiperspirants. Some of these contain toxic chemicals. Even those that claim to be "natural" clog the pores of the underarm lymph glands and prevent the body from releasing toxic substances. When the body is over-whelmed with toxins from the air, water, drugs and foods, often the main detoxifying systems (the liver, kidneys and lungs) can no longer excrete the load. The body then uses an auxiliary sys-tem—perspiration—to help detoxify.

Unfortunately, this toxic excretion in perspiration is smelly. Naturally, people have been educated to use a deodorant cream or stick to help prevent undesirable odor. However, using deodorants blocks the lymph glands and propels toxins back into the lymph system of the breast and underarm. It is even likely that male breast cancer, which is increasing considerably, is directly related to the use of deodorants.

It is, admittedly, difficult in our "civilized, industrial society" to avoid all these harmful factors. And cancer, particularly the glandular cancer that affects the breast, can take months or years to appear. Once it is diagnosed, however, it is imperative to eliminate all toxins to aid the healing process.

The second major factor in all malignancies is deficiency of our depleted and artificially fertilized soil that does not produce food rich in natural nutrients. The food is further depleted, as we have discussed, through being refined and treated in process-ing such as jarring, canning, freezing and preparing for its dis-pensing as "fast foods."

Gerson's Therapy treats the cancer patient's severely toxic and deficient body that loses its natural immunity, hormone bal-ance, enzyme activity and ability to handle stress and/or acci-dents or injuries. Of course, the therapy's success depends on how exactly and consistently it is carried out over a suitably long period of time. Admittedly, this is a difficult, expensive process, needing much help and support from the patient's care-givers. Any variation or omission can endanger the good out-come; so can the patient's unwillingness to work wholeheartedly and in a positive frame of mind for his or her recovery.

And there are many factors that can prevent healing. The most common cause of failure is that patients come to the therapy far too late: in terminal condition, most often having vainly tried to recover on conventional treatments, especially on highly toxic chemotherapy, which destroys the patients' remaining, already badly damaged immune system. Once the organism has declined beyond a certain point, there is no way to restore it.

A system of detoxification

In addition to powerfully supporting the cancer patient's body with a strict dietary regimen that required a high degree of compliance from the patient and close supervision and frequent adjustment by the physician, Gerson perfected a system of detoxing the body as well.

He believed that the digestive tracts of late-stage cancer patients were extremely poisoned with cancer. The liver and pancreas fail to function and nothing is alive. To stimulate the liver, he administered frequent coffee enemas as well as castor oil by mouth and as an enema,[17] which was not uncommon treatment at the time.[18]

Although these enemas were used primarily to help the cancerous body excrete toxic wastes, especially from dying tumors, researchers now realize that these enemas also aid the body in absorbing vitamin A.[19] As we saw, vitamin A represents a vital component of Gerson's treatment. Vitamin A plays an essential role in supporting immune function.[20] The coffee enemas also reduce pain, which patients found very helpful since Gerson's treatment avoids the use of painkillers and any other drugs that might overtax the liver.

Eventually this brilliant scientist added iodine to the treatment regimen as well, because of its abilities in supporting the immune system, after he discovered that it seemed to counteract the cancer-causing effects of hormones.[21]

Medical community reaction—1950s

Although Dr. Gerson's research was powerful, well documented and quite complete, the medical establishment largely bypassed or overlooked it. As we have discussed, conventional medical scientists still viewed cancer in terms of a tumor that needed to be excised, not as a systemic or whole body disease.

Two thousand years ago, ancient Chinese writings observed that an immoderate diet increased the risk for disease of the esophagus. Yet in the 1950s, the American Medical Association and American Cancer Society denounced Dr. Max Gerson, along with other outstanding physicians, for using nutrition as part of a comprehensive treatment for cancer.

It didn't help Gerson's cause that he came out very strongly against tobacco in a time when Phillip Morris was the major source of advertising revenue for the American Medical Association's prestigious and influential magazine, *Journal of the American Medical Association*.[22]

Sadly, the years of research and a good response from 30 percent of his cancer patients[23] were swept aside in an ensuing wave of politics. Funding that might have gone toward additional research into dietary treatments for cancer was poured into drug research.

The medical community's initiative—1980s

Then, in the 1980s, the American Cancer Society issued dietary guidelines for reducing the risk of developing cancer, a diet remarkably similar to the Gerson diet.[24] In 1982, the congressionally appointed panel of the National Academy of Sciences released their book *Diet, Nutrition, and Cancer*, in which they stated boldly: "Spread the good news that cancer is not as inevitable as death and taxes."

Now cancer authorities readily admit that some 50–55 percent of women's cancers are caused by faulty nutrition. And while the *Journal of the American Medical Association* in the 1930s advertised cigarettes—"20,679 physicians say 'Luckies' are less irritating"—

they now point not only to smoking but also to breathing second-hand smoke as a contributing to causing cancer.

Living proof that "it works!"

In the course of the past decade, a great deal of cancer research has shown that certain food factors help to inhibit the spreading and growth of malignancies. In a new book called *Living Proof: A Medical Mutiny*, Michael Gearin-Tosch describes his own survival of multiple myeloma without conventional treatment of chemotherapy. He was treated mainly with the Gerson Therapy. While the orthodox authorities in Great Britain and in the United States gave him 0.005 percent chance of recovering without chemotherapy, he chose, nevertheless, to follow the natural healing system. He is surviving and living an active life eight years beyond his cancer diagnosis.

A contributor to the book, Dr. Carmen Wheatley, who is a respected researcher (not a medical doctor), discusses some of the nutritional factors of the Gerson Therapy:

- Fresh fruit, particularly apples, contain a chemical called quercetin, known to "promote cell death" of cancer tissue. Quercetin is referred to by Dr. Patrick Quillan of the Cancer Treatment Centers of America as "one of the most potent anticarcinogens in nature."[25]

- The Gerson Therapy is very rich in isocyanates from cruciferous vegetables such as cabbage, broccoli and beets.

- It is also rich in allium (from garlic), a natural detoxifier, and in selenium (from onion, leeks, scallions and chives). Selenium and allium have been shown to enhance DNA repair.

- Further, the Gerson Therapy contains the Omega-3 fatty acids (from linseed oil), which interfere with metastasis and also promote the death of diseased cells.

It is important to note that Dr. T. Colin Campbell, professor of nutrition at Cornell University, has shown in long-term experiments that artificially produced nutrients (he used beta carotene) do not have the same positive effect as the natural elements found in carrots. They provided no protection, much less healing activity. Again, living food is the ultimate source for nutrient protection against disease.

In the present climate, where people have been conditioned to expect "a pill for every ill" and not take responsibility for their own health, the Gerson Therapy may seem to be a difficult path to follow. But when it comes to saving one's life and building a healthy future, the effort is certainly worthwhile.

Dr. Max Gerson, a revolutionary scientist who pioneered his "radical" discoveries early in the twentieth century, had learned empirically that food has physical and chemical qualities that heal. Forty years later, another kind of pioneer motivated a movement of people to seek physical and spiritual health through nutritional methods.

(The author would like to thank Charlotte Gerson, daughter of Dr. Max Gerson, for her kind contribution of much of the above material regarding her father's medical work.)

A Reverend Promotes Diet Therapy

In the spring of 1976, Reverend George Malkmus began experiencing a feeling of pressure under his left rib cage—not pain, just pressure. Tests revealed a cancerous tumor the size of a baseball in his colon where the transverse and descending colon pocket together. This news was especially terrifying to Malkmus since his mother had recently died of colon cancer. According to Malkmus, his mother who was a registered nurse, had been a vital and hearty woman.

Shortly after medical treatments, which included surgery,

chemotherapy and radiation for her cancer, her health began to deteriorate at a terrifying rate. Watching his mother weaken and expire, Malkmus became convinced that it was the treatment, not the cancer, that caused her death. This tragic experience was sobering, and Malkmus determined never to take his mother's route. He made this decision despite the fact that as a nurse she had taught her son to follow carefully and faithfully medical advice.

Malkmus needed an alternative for the conventional cancer treatment his mother had taken, so he began a search. He remembered another minister who had been severely criticized as a "health nut" by his peers in ministry. This pastor suggested that Malkmus completely change his normal American diet of meat and potatoes with plenty of sugary sweets for dessert and begin to eat an all-raw vegetarian diet with lots of carrot juice.

Having no other recourse, Malkmus took the plunge. Within days of following this radical new diet, he felt much worse. His body had begun a natural process of detoxification, which caused him to feel poorly while the body was expelling years of built-up waste. But after a few weeks the cleansing reactions abated, and he started to feel better than he had in years.

In less than one year on a raw-food diet and drinking one to two quarts of carrot juice a day, Reverend Malkmus's cancer tumor totally disappeared. But that's not all. Not only had his tumor completely disappeared, but other more minor physical problems he had been experiencing were gone, too. These included allergies, fatigue, high blood pressure, hypoglycemia, hemorrhoids, acne and even body odor and dandruff—it appeared that the radical diet had purged his entire body of disease.

The good pastor has been on a modified version of this vegetarian diet since then and has never experienced a recurrence of cancer or any other sickness. Almost thirty years later, his diet still consists of 85 percent raw vegetables and fruits (no more than 15 percent fruit) and 15 percent cooked vegetables. The cooked vegetables include baked potatoes, steamed vegetables, brown rice, baked squash, sweet potatoes and occasionally whole-grain pastas. He also has 3 to 4 tablespoons of Barley Green in a daily drink.

Malkmus claims that on this diet, which he dubbed the Hallelujah Diet, he has not experienced so much as a cold or needed to take any medication, not even an aspirin, in nearly thirty years. He also claims that his physical abilities, stamina, energy and endurance are better than when he was a teenager.[26]

Malkmus never pretended to hold any of the trappings of the scientific establishment; he was neither a scientist nor a physician. He was simply a man with cancer who cured himself by drastically changing his own diet. He didn't discover anything new, but simply took advantage of widely published information, which he later realized had been available in the Bible for centuries. He was able to influence many people to do the same.

Both Gerson and Malkmus, men of different generations with widely divergent backgrounds and very different educations, stumbled upon the same scientific truth that produced healing. Gerson, a scientist, demonstrated empirically that food has physical and chemical qualities that heal. Malkmus cured himself with foods and found that the Bible contained information pointing to this truth all along. Their experiences have a very scientific validation.

A Scientific Factor for Dietary Treatment

As we discussed, Warburg discovered that the malignant cell is anaerobe or partially anaerobe, meaning that cancers do not do well in the oxygen-rich environment that the rest of our cells need to be at their best. This discovery that the metabolism of cancer cells were quite different from normal cells was a breakthrough of epic proportions that the scientific community had overlooked.

But what does the oxygen factor have to do with the dietary treatment of cancer? A lot! You may have studied the Krebs cycle in your high school biology class, that process through which our cells obtain energy (adenosine triphosphate, ATP) by metabolizing carbohydrates. This most vital metabolic process cannot happen in the absence of oxygen. People who die from drowning do not die just because oxygen did not get to their lungs; they die because their cells could not produce ATP, especially in the brain.

Malignant cells also need ATP to survive, though they do not tolerate oxygen. So how do they get the ATP they need in an oxygen-poor environment? They have to "burn" protein or fat to obtain ATP. Burning protein and fat results in the production of lactic acid, a harmful toxic waste difficult to excrete. These chemical reactions pull sodium into the cell and displace the potassium from within the cell, which changes the electrical polarity of the cell.

If you eat only a vegetarian diet that consists of carbohydrates, you avoid burning protein and fat and the resultant destructive chemical reactions. This diet of carbohydrates actually "starves" the cancer cell, which is why Malkmus and some of Dr. Gerson's patients were able to cure themselves of cancer.

Obviously, it is not always so simple to rid yourself of cancer. Malignant cells are quite resourceful and will find alternate sources of protein and fat. Unfortunately, they do not have to look far. Next to water, protein and fat are the

> We need always to remember that we treat patients, not diseases.

most common elements in our body. Still, whatever you can do through diet to complicate the malignant cell's life will be greatly appreciated by your immune system. For example, if you consume little or no added salt to your diet, the malignant cell, which must draw sodium into it to maintain its antipolarity, will suffer even more.

Dietary Treatment at the Oasis of Hope

Physicians and healers should understand that not everything orthodox is bad and not all alternatives are good. We need always to remember that we treat patients, not diseases. What this means is that no matter what is ailing the patient, his or her needs are singularly their own. That is why there is no therapy or even diet that is good for everyone.

As a general rule I propose that you eat the living foods the Bible teaches us to eat in the Old Testament. It will also be beneficial to eat these foods as close to the original state in which God created them as possible. For example, raw fruits and vegetables are the most nutritious forms of these foods. In the next chapter we discuss how most of the foods God chose for mankind have been adulterated and nutritionally devalued through industrial manipulation to the point that much of it has become deleterious to our health. We cannot simply eat what tastes good or what our culture has offered us.

> **Physicians and healers should understand that not everything orthodox is bad and not all alternatives are good.**

A Cancer-Free Future

The Bible declares, "And you shall know the truth, and the truth shall make you free" (John 8:32, NKJV). Because we do not yet know the whole truth about cancer, we do not understand all of its causes. And its ultimate cure continues to elude us. But it is gradually giving up its secret destructive patterns to persistent and open-minded research. We have learned much about the complicated puzzle behind this disease.

We now know that a great part of the coming cure for cancer rests in diet and dietary research. Diet holds a key to treatment, but the power of a dietary solution certainly doesn't stop there. The American Cancer Society, which publishes national statistics on cancer every year, boldly proclaims that cancer can be completely beaten even in our lifetime. The reason they can declare that promise is that they now know almost all cancer can be *prevented*. In order to experience the prevention of cancer, we must begin to embrace the truth of proper diet in our lives and the lives of our families—and future generations.

The most powerful way to attack cancer is to determine to build and maintain a healthy body, mind and spirit—that is what we call *prevention*. Preventive medicine is being aggressively pursued on many fronts. It needs to be understood and become the treatment of choice for millions who do not want to succumb to the ravages of cancer.

Section III

Promoting Prevention

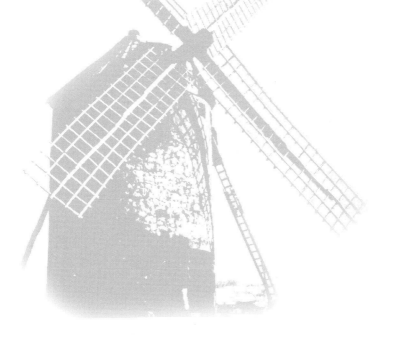

8 The Power of Prevention— Living Foods

I n 1927, following the complaints of a forty-two-year-old woman, Drs. Chalk and Foucar of the Ontario Hospital, Canada, examined her and removed 2,533 objects, including 947 bent pins, from her stomach. Two hundred twelve objects were removed from the stomach of a man admitted to Groote Schuur Hospital, Cape Town, South Africa in May 1985. The objects included fifty-three toothbrushes, two telescopic aerials, two razors and one hundred fifty handles of disposable razors.[1] Records show that another man ground up and pulverized a bus over the period of several years and ate the entire vehicle! These eccentric individuals inadvertently proved the resilience of the human body to ingested abuse.

The typical American diet is far more nourishing than the eccentric diets of these unfortunate individuals. Or is it? Think about your last trip to the local convenience store. You encountered a great deal of expensive food there for sale, but what nourishment did it offer? There were aisles and aisles of shiny packages of processed fatty, sugary items of various shapes, sizes and often amazingly unnatural colors. These "food" items included gooey pastries, orange and pink powdery chips and bright-blue drinks that are visually indistinguishable from commercial toilet cleaners located in the next aisle.

Perhaps you moved on to another shelf. Crossing over to the

refrigerator section you found frosty pre-made sandwiches waiting for you, made with sticky, devitalized white bread that could wrap around your incisors like Super Glue, leaving you digging and scraping your teeth in order to talk. Ugh!

Well, there was a shiny red apple on the counter! But it had been radiated to give it a far longer shelf life—leaving barely enough vitamins and minerals to make crunching through the waxy pesticide coating worthwhile.

What has become of our food supply? Where is the vital nourishment that God originally intended for us when He said to Adam and Eve, "Behold, I have given you every plant yielding seed that is on the surface of all the earth, and every tree which has fruit yielding seed; it shall be food for you" (Gen. 1:29). Sadly, in terms of nutritional value, much of today's food bears greater resemblance to the eccentric diets of pins and screws of the abovementioned individuals than it does to the diet originally envisioned for us by our Creator.

We possess an enormous power over cancer—possibly enough to eradicate it completely—through prevention. Prevention is the most powerful tool we have with which to fight every disease and preserve life. The preservation of God's gift of health is, I'm convinced, a moral duty. To fulfill that duty it is vital that every individual become informed regarding the level of living nutrition the food they eat is actually giving to them.

The Food Industry

Until the end of the nineteenth century, most people lived off the land and depended upon a very restricted and monotonous seasonal diet yielded by the crops of that season. Food was cultivated, gathered, cooked and then eaten. There was little means of storing foods for any length of time. That changed dramatically when the Industrial Revolution brought greater productivity of crops as well as new methods to preserve food.

Now the United States produces enough food to feed the entire world's population. Yet much of the world continues to experience famine. Why? It is true that wars, droughts, floods and other natural factors ruin foodstuffs. But the ugly reality is that politics and economics are the real agricultural assassins. Food is destroyed or stored to maintain its high market value so that even when it is available, people around the globe cannot afford to purchase the food they need.

While food is out of reach economically for millions, millions more in the world's industrialized countries overeat and waste their abundant food supply. Added to that is the sad reality that the birth of the food industry has resulted in giving us food that is increasingly mechanized, electrified, fertilized, "pesticised," sterilized, refined and processed. These devitalized foods, even in lands of plenty, give far less actual nourishment than the foods from an earlier century did.

Helping Mother Nature

Today agriculture is a multibillion-dollar business. Years ago we produced food to survive, and now we produce food to make money—lots of it. Modern agriculture has become a lucrative and creative industry, ever on the lookout for ways to become even more profitable. One doesn't need to search very far to discover how increased productivity affects profit in the food business. Many increase productivity by manipulating nature with chemical fertilizers to shorten the harvest time and pesticides to diminish losses. Others increase profit by distributing the product at a time when the best prices can be obtained instead of shortly after harvest when nutrients are the highest.

But the best way industry giants have found to increase profit is to actually transform perishable food into imperishable food. What is frightening is the fact that these methods used to increase productivity and profit also severely damage the nutritional value of the food produced. And in many cases, the nutritional value is virtually erased.

Foods grown today are processed with three objectives: to be tasty, precooked and imperishable (indestructible). In other words, these imperishable foods can stay on your shelf or in your refrigerator for months (and sometimes for years) and still be edible. These "high-profit" foods are the backbone of the food industry. They are presented in shiny, appealing packages and have an endless shelf life. But what consumers are missing is that the reason these foods last so long is because they have little more nutritional value than the pretty box they come in.

Hunger in the affluent societies of the world is tastefully, conveniently and artificially answered by the food industry. The fastest-growing companies within the food industry are fast (processed, precooked) food corporations. Throughout the world fast-food restaurants are continually opening. And the food industry spends millions to increase demand and consumption for its products.

But our bodies are crying out for nutritious food to meet the challenges of a modern existence that subjects us to the threat of cancer and a host of other degenerative diseases. Contrary to popular beliefs, eating is not just a recreational activity. It should be an area of great concern on which we focus our attention to assure that we get the nutrients we need for health.

Most of us don't spend a great deal of time considering the nutritional quality of the foods we consume. For many individuals, this can be a fatal mistake. The fast foods creatively produced to save us minutes in our days steal years from our lives.

Wanted: Fruits and vegetables—dead or alive!

We don't need a Ph.D. in nutrition to understand that the Creator's design for eating involves a more important goal than satisfying our taste buds. We know intuitively and then by experience that we have to refuel our bodies regularly with energy in order to function normally.

It's interesting to me that ancient cultures from all parts of the world seemed to provide the nutrients necessary to maintain health even though the "raw materials" for their diets were so different from each other. Various cultures developed their own distinctive culinary art. Yet each recipe represents a treatise in biochemistry.

I doubt that our ancestors spent much time considering the biochemical reactions they produced in their kitchens. But somehow they knew what was needed and what satisfied the requirements of nutrition for health—as well as those of their taste buds. Yet, it is so easy for us to forget that the foods we eat

> # The fast foods creatively produced to save us minutes in our days steal years from our lives.

are primarily a vehicle for transporting the nutrients that generate the energy our bodies require.

Almost all of these vital nutrients come from the ground. The easiest way to transport these vital nutrients from the soil to our bodies where they provide the fuel we need is by eating living foods such as fruits and vegetables. But alive, fresh foods are perishable and easily attacked by a wide variety of natural elements, from pests to decomposition. That fact created big problems for a food industry—problems that called for creative (though not always nutritious) solutions.

That's why manufactures determined that we would be just as satisfied to have our produce dead as alive. One of the ways they alter fresh produce is through chemical chaos.

Awash in chemical chaos. Farmers wage an endless war against the pests that attack living foods. An entire chemical industry has developed to destroy these pesky little critters. War against them is waged with various kinds of pesticides in order to "protect" the consumer. But the truth is that farmers are protecting their crop from being eaten by the bugs. These bugs are harmless to consumers and are easily eliminated if they wash produce carefully.

Fertilizers are another chemical mainstay of the food industry that our ancestors would have known nothing about. Vast amounts of poisonous chemical fertilizers are dumped into the soil to increase the yield of crops—crops that are often then destroyed or warehoused in order to keep food prices high. This chemical abuse of our soil through the excessive use of fertilizers and pesticides erodes and strips it of its nutrients. Consequently, the nutritional value of the fruits and vegetables produced from such soil is dramatically diminished.

The law of God. We have broken God's laws in respect to our soil, and we are reaping the consequences. He instructed Moses specifically to care for the earth as early as 1490 B.C.:

> Six years you shall sow your field, and six years you shall prune your vineyard and gather in its crop, but during the seventh year the land shall have a sabbath rest, a sabbath to the LORD; you shall not sow your field nor prune your vineyard. Your harvest's aftergrowth you shall not reap, and your grapes of untrimmed vines you shall not gather; the land shall have a sabbatical year.
>
> —LEVITICUS 25:3–5

For centuries folk wisdom adhered to this law of rest for the land, and the land produced bountiful crops that were packed with health-producing vital nutrients, minerals, enzymes and amino acids. The wisdom of God to allow the land to replenish itself every seventh year maintained its vitality.

Nutrients destroyed; poisons added. Today, not only is the land overused and depleted, but the most frequently used fertilizers destroy iron, vitamin C, folic acid, minerals, lysine, amino acids and many other nutrients. Pesticides contaminate the soil and take a long time to disappear. For example, chlordane has a half-life of twenty years. That means that in twenty years, it will still be half as strong as it was when applied to the soil.

Remember that all plants absorb the substances found in the earth in which they grow. While authorities have prohibited the use of pesticides that have been proven to be strong carcinogens, the weak carcinogenic pesticides are still considered safe (only to a scientist paid by the pesticide industry!). The problem is that in the laboratories they are tested individually. But in real life they are never used alone. These chemicals are combined with others, which dramatically increases their cancer-causing effects.

Pesticides contaminate more than 94 percent of the foods we eat. Without a doubt, continuous exposure to them can cause cancer and other degenerative diseases. In 1968, a research group found that patients who died from liver cancer, brain cancer, multiple sclerosis and other degenerative diseases had significantly higher traces of pesticides in their brains and fatty tissue than those who had died from other diseases.[2]

Some of the pesticides considered less toxic can still cause depression, migraines, hyperactivity and more. Pesticides are easily absorbed and hard to eliminate; they remain in our body with dire effects because of their chemical affinity to estrogen (as we will discuss later).

"Incorruptible" produce. A couple of years ago, a family friend purchased their traditional pumpkin for the harvest season. After Thanksgiving, they placed it in their garage where it sat—and sat. It seemed it would never spoil. For months they kept checking it, wondering how much longer the "super" pumpkin would last. It became a little game.

Finally, several months later it was thrown into the trash, more out of boredom than because it had yielded to the corruption of all living things. It might still be sitting there today—two years later—had it not been thrown away. It may well be sitting at the dump looking the same today as it did then. My friend concluded that the tennis racket leaning on the wall next to the pumpkin would have decayed sooner.

What makes bacteria thrive? To realize the negative impact of this incorruptible produce on our bodies, we need to understand what makes food rot and biodegrade. The answer to that question is nothing more or less than bacterial invasion—when bacteria start eating the food, the food rots. In other words, bacteria feed on the same nutrients our bodies need to survive. If there are no nutrients in the food or there are poisons present, bacteria stay away and the food does not rot.

Do you get the picture? Even bacteria won't "eat" devitalized or poisoned food. Should you? Conversely, if bacteria beat you to the food, you know it was free of poisons and rich in nutrients; it was edible.

My friends' immortal pumpkin must have been radiated, which is another way that the food industry is manipulating our food, causing bacteria to leave it alone. With the help of modern technology, the food industry has learned to use radiation to sanitize produce, which increases profits by prolonging shelf life. However, these radioisotopes not only destroy nutrients in produce, but their particles easily enter into our living cells where they increase the risk of cell mutation and cancer.

Times have changed. Not many years ago, our fruit selections were dependent upon the seasons in which they grew. But those days of eating strawberries in the spring and apples in the fall are over. Today, we can have the kind of produce we want when we want it, thanks to the radiation process. Increased consumer demands require efficient management of soil, early harvesting techniques, storage, packaging and transportation of foods. Unfortunately, this accelerated produce production in nutrient-deprived soil creates nutritionally depleted vegetables and fruits. Add the radiation process to these compromised foods, and the nutritional picture is even bleaker.

What bugs know about wheat

In the same way that bacteria know what kinds of food they need to eat to thrive, insects seem to know something about what you're eating that you may not.

For many generations, wheat was the staff of life for cultures around the world. It supplied a rich and wonderful source of protein, amino acids, complex carbohydrates and fiber. Today, about 360 million metric tons of wheat are harvested worldwide each year.

But our bodies no longer benefit from this wonderful natural product. Wheat too was handed a death sentence by the food processors. The wheat we eat today has been completely devitalized, stripped of its nutrients and its ability to nourish the body.

Refining wheat has turned it into another dead food. You no longer need to worry about how long it's been sitting on your pantry shelf. You won't find bugs in your flour or your bread—there's not enough nutrition in it to attract a bug! In this respect, bugs may be smarter than we are; they refuse to eat what doesn't nourish them.

The flour you eat is as dead as the ground-up bus eaten by the man we mentioned earlier. When wheat is refined it loses:

- 80 percent of its vitamin B_1 (thiamin)
- 80 percent of its B_2 (riboflavin)
- 80 percent of its B_3 (niacin) and B_6
- 98 percent of its vitamin E
- 90 percent of its minerals and micronutrients
- 80 percent of its biotin
- 76 percent of its vitamin K
- 75 percent of its folic acid
- 50 percent of its linoleic acid
- 99 percent of its fiber
- 100 percent of about twenty-seven other nutrients

The only benefit of refining wheat is that it increases its caloric value by 7 percent!

Appearance is everything!

Another consideration of the food industry is that the average consumer demands produce that "looks" good. To protect produce from dents, scrapes and bruises, vegetables and fruits are specially boxed or piled. This is done in spite of the fact that when picked and left outside more than two or three hours, their nutritional value is reduced by 40 to 50 percent.

Potatoes lose up to 78 percent of their vitamin C a week after they are harvested; spinach greens, asparagus, broccoli and peas lose 50 percent of their vitamins before they ever get to market. Packaging and transportation of produce compromises nutritional value even more. And produce sitting in storage loses additional nutrients.

To increase shelf life and appearance, farmers harvest their fruits and vegetables long before they are mature. That may seem innocent enough, for we have gradually lowered our expectations regarding flavor. But fruits and vegetables absorb most of their vitamins and minerals when they are almost ripe. The next time you pick up a bunch of bright, green bananas, think about this: They will never fill up with the vitamins and minerals they would have acquired ripening in the sun by sitting on supermarket shelves or on your kitchen counters! So once again nutrition takes a back seat—this time to appearance. Unfortunately, appearance may be just about all this deficient produce gives you.

The wonders of processed foods

Processed foods are even more profitable than manipulated produce simply because they last longer. Availability and convenience move the industry to provide imperishable user-friendly foods to the consumer in cans, cartons or frozen bags. But, in every step of the process, vital nutrients are sacrificed.

Juices and milk are usually packaged in carton containers lined with wax, a known cancer-causing substance. Plastic containers aren't much better since they are made from petrochemicals (polymers with toxic stabilizers and color tinctures like acrylic acid), tuolene, Styrofoam and vinyl chloride. These carcinogens, or cancer-causing agents, abound in disposable plates, bowls and cups as well.

Most frozen vegetables lose 25 percent of vitamins A, B_1, B_2, C and niacin, among others, during the process of freezing. Broccoli, cauliflower, peas and spinach lose up to 50 percent of vitamins as a result of freezing.

Canned foods lose more than 50 percent of all nutrients due

to the canning process. In addition, nitrites, which are added to kill botulism, when heated with the food are converted into nitrosamines, another potent cancer-causing substance.

By the time these "new tech" foods get to our mouths, they have already been through a chamber of food "tortures." They have been sprayed with acidifiers, alkalinizers, antifoaming agents, artificial colors, artificial flavors, sweeteners, deodorants, fillers, disinfectants, emulsifiers, extenders, hydrogenators, moisturizers and plenty more. As a final insult, they are given a lash with synthetic vitamins to replace chemically what has been lost!

No wonder bacteria will not touch the stuff! These modern and profit-making foods are so "well made" that they are practically indestructible.

The preservatives prowess

Unobstructed by authorities, backed by investors, encouraged by profits and waved on by our ignorance, food producers have raced down the path of chemical chaos, adding ever-increasing amounts of preservatives to our foods. In the 1960s Americans consumed about three pounds per person per year of these noxious chemicals, in the seventies about six pounds,[3] and since then we have crossed the ten-pound line.

Curiously, health officials are not alarmed by the increase in morbidity and mortality caused by fast and convenient *un*-foods. Morticians, however, are astonished to find corpses that long ago should have been converted to ashes still as fresh as a newly picked lettuce! They report that the average time for a cadaver to decompose today is twice as long as thirty years ago. What a phenomenon! Food preservatives that accelerate our trip to the grave give us the macabre advantage of keeping us presentable longer in our tombs! If only the pharaohs knew.

What about the sacred cow?

Ever since cowboys sat around crackling campfires at night

singing "Home on the Range" to their mooing steer, Americans have loved meat. The demand for beef and other meats has steadily increased through the years. To supply this enormous demand, the food industry has developed scientific methods to increase the production of red and white meats.

In 1940 more than four pounds of feed were needed to produce one pound of meat. In the 1980s, only two pounds were required.[4] Fifty years ago, a cow produced two thousand pounds of milk per year. Presently, milk producers get fifty thousand pounds of milk per year per cow.[5] How have such marvelous increases in production been achieved? Through chemically enhanced feeds, genetic engineering, drugs and hormones the modern livestock industry has created super chickens and monster cows.

Consumers now have access to the information about most of what they are ingesting, thanks to recent FDA labeling regulations. But, despite strong complaints, livestock producers have had preferential treatment and are not required to list the additives and ingredients in their products. This leaves consumers to surmise that meat is purely meat, and milk is…well, milk. Right?

Actually, the FDA allows the administration of up to eighty-two drugs to cows in the production of dairy products.[6] Among these drugs, the bovine growth hormone and estrogen are the most abused. Of all the drugs used to fatten livestock and tenderize their meat, the most harmful to humans is the female hormone estrogen.

Scientific research suggests that the effects of bovine growth hormone and estrogen together on the body can cause arthritis, obesity, glucose intolerance, diabetes and heart disease. They may also be responsible for other less serious but annoying maladies, including headaches, fatigue, vision impairment, dizziness, menstrual problems and loss of sexual drive.[7]

Let me hasten to say that meat and milk are not bad for you; otherwise God would not have recommended them in our diet. What has become a menace to our health is their profitable adulteration by the food industry. But fortunately more and more organically produced meat and milk are being made available.

A closer look at estrogen contamination

The harmful effects I listed above caused by estrogen and estrogen-like substances account for much of the modern malaise of "dis-ease." As I mentioned previously, just about all our foods contain pesticides. Most of these pesticides have a chemical structure very closely related to estrogen—close enough to fool our bodies. When we eat pesticide-tainted foods, they provoke a weak estrogenic effect on our systems.

The plastics that wrap and keep our foods fresh also mildly behave like estrogen in our bodies. Since the hormonal effects of such materials are weak, we consider such products safe. But when so many of the materials and foods around us have been tainted, the compounded effect is strengthened significantly. The consequences of the combined estrogenic effect of all of these products can be powerful.

An example of the strength of this estrogen imitation is the livestock contamination that occurred on a Michigan farm. Here the livestock feed was contaminated with the pesticide Polychlorinated Biphenyl (PCB), which is considered a "weak" estrogen imitator. However, pregnant women and mothers who consumed the meat of these animals and then breast-fed their children were horrified to find that their male children developed genital deformities and very small penises.[8]

In Taiwan, Chinese scientists have under observation 118 male children of mothers who were contaminated with PCB in an accidental spill in 1989. These boys suffer from the same painful complications as the boys from the Michigan farm contamination.[9]

In lakes with high concentrations of DDT and DDE—pesticides that also have estrogenic effects—the fauna have been severely degenerated. Alligators of Lake Apopka in Florida have lost virility because of low testosterone and sperm count; the sizes of their male organs are one-fourth smaller than the norm. The Great Lakes are gravely polluted with PCB and DDT; the result is that many fish and seagulls that get their food there have developed grotesque hormonal dysfunction that make them hermaphrodite, according to Theo Colburn of the World Wildlife Fund.[10]

Niels Skakkebaek, a Danish endocrinologist and probably the foremost authority on the subject of estrogen, reported in 1991 that because of the exaggerated exposure to estrogen and estrogen-like substances, men presently have only 50 percent of the normal sperm count. They also are experiencing a significant reduction in the size of their reproductive organs, and the incidence of testicular cancer has tripled.[11]

These chemicals have mercilessly maimed our society's virility, sex drive, fatherhood and manhood. Synthetic estrogens and the chemical agents that mimic estrogen represent a very real threat to health. They do not breakdown easily, and our bodies cannot neutralize them. They end up tainting our entire food chain and remain active for many years.

Long Island, New York has one of the highest incidence of breast cancer in the United States. Experts believe this is due to the vast quantity of pesticides used on the farming soils before they were converted to urban communities. Today, these pesticides are still abundant in the local tap water.[12]

Mary Wolf, M.D., a professor at Mt. Sinai School of Medicine in New York, reported that breast tumor biopsies of women from Long Island showed unusually high concentrations of DDT and DDE. And the incidence of cancer was four times higher than in biopsies where the pesticides are absent or in low concentrations.[13] Research overwhelmingly supports that estrogen increases the incidence of many female ailments, including cancer of the breast, uterus and ovaries.

Cancer is only one of the many ailments that estrogens have brought upon women. Menstrual, fertility, ovarian and uterine problems can also be listed. German scientists have discovered high blood concentrations of PCB in women suffering with endometriosis, an inflammatory pelvic disease that causes severe pain and sterility. Before pesticides arrived on the scene, endometriosis was virtually unheard of. In 1920, only twenty-one cases had been reported worldwide. Today, upwards of five million women battle this painful problem in the United States alone!

The nightmare of nitrates

Purchasing gray or brown meat from the butcher's section of your favorite grocer would probably not be very appealing. If you are like most shoppers, you look for bright red meat as an indicator of freshness. You may already be aware that the red color doesn't suggest freshness anymore. Today's meat is packed with nitrates to give it the red color we equate with freshness when we select hamburger or steak.

Nitrates, a pillar of the meat industry, become a serious cancer-causing agent when heated. Nitrates are also widely used in the preparation of lunch meats, hot dogs and bacon. It's been shown that children who eat twelve or more hot dogs a month are 9.5 times as likely to get leukemia.[14] When pregnant mothers eat hot dogs during pregnancy, the incidence of brain cancer in their children increases dramatically as well.[15]

One of the only truly natural things left in our meat is the fat—and there's plenty of that. Nearly 60 percent of meat and dairy products, including milk, eggs, cheese and processed meats, is fat. The fatty meats and dairy products we consume tend to trap the toxic chemicals and antibiotics, dramatically increasing our risk of obesity, hypertension, cardiovascular diseases, hyperthyroidism, candidiasis and cancer. Of the one hundred forty-three chemical substances found in commercial meats, forty-two are cancer causing or carcinogenic, and twenty more can cause birth defects.[16]

Vegetable oils unmasked

Animal fats have been considered so harmful that health experts began to recommend the consumption of vegetable oils instead. These oils are obtained from grains, seeds and nuts. For centuries vegetable oils have been used around the world for nutritional, medicinal and religious purposes. Through simple compression of the plants or grains you can obtain excellent quality oils.

However, because they also contain an enormous amount of nutrients, these natural vegetable oils tend to spoil very quickly; they are also very appealing to bacteria. Therefore, to increase the shelf life of vegetable oil, experts developed a process called mechanical extraction. In this process pressure mills crush the seeds and then heat the mash to 240 degrees. Afterward, the unrefined oil is pressed at over twenty tons of pressure per square inch. This removes from the oil all the elements that can spoil. Unfortunately, all the nutritional value is also lost. Today's vegetable oils have no more nutritional value than the motor oil in your car has.

To create a less-expensive process for extracting oil from grains, scientists produced a chemical extraction method. In this method, seeds are heated to 160 degrees, and then they are allowed to rest in gasoline, hexane, ethylene, carbon disulfide, tetrachloride or methyl chloride. Afterward, the solvent is evaporated, though a very minute portion remains mixed with the oil. Then the carotene is removed through a chlorination process, yielding crystal-clear oil.

Although this process is able to extend the shelf life almost indefinitely, it also destroys any nutritional value. Even worse it makes the fatty acids toxic. Margarine and vegetable shortening are hydrogenated and made solid by high pressure and heating the oil to 380 degrees. Our bodies cannot metabolize these substances, which also hinder them from using other oils they need.

Fake fats

In January 1996, the Food and Drug Administration gave Proctor and Gamble permission to sell snack foods, such as chips, fried in Olean (the trademark of Olestra, which is a fake fat). Olean is a proven anti-nutrient. In other words, not only does it not give anything to your body that is nutritious, but it actually robs nutrition from the body.

Olean is designed to look and taste like fat, but unlike fat, it cannot be absorbed into the body from the intestinal tract. It runs freely through your gastrointestinal tract unabsorbed and is passed out in the feces. It may cause anal leakage, and as fat passes through the intestines unabsorbed, fat-soluble nutrients attach to it and are carried out also. Among these fat-soluble nutrients that are lost are beta carotene, a cancer fighter, and other carotenoids. Studies reveal that upwards of 40 percent of carotenoids may be reduced by eating Olean.[17]

Fake diet foods such as Olean do not actually reduce obesity. In fact, the opposite is true; they have been linked to weight gain.

A Nutrient Death Sentence

Many of the foods you eat were handed a nutritional death sentence by the food processing industry. Refined sugar, refined flour and processed oils make up the core of this industry. They cost almost nothing to produce, they last forever on the shelf, and they are the primary ingredients in all processed foods.

Sugar was the first food to receive the deathblow against its nutritional value. About two hundred years ago profiteers discovered they could "purify" sugar of any elements that might cause it to decompose without taking away its sweetness. They called the process required to purify sugar *refining*.

Refining sugar strips it entirely of its nutritional value, creating naked calories. Refined sugar is composed of 96 percent sucrose, 3 percent waste, 1 percent water and 0 percent nutrition. Another example of "naked calories" is corn syrup. Corn syrup is also an "anti-nutrient." It not only has zero nutritional value, but it also robs the body of nutrients such as thiamin, riboflavin and niacin.

Since its advent in 1751, refined sugar has been the most consumed food stock worldwide. We start taking in refined sugar almost from birth. As a matter of fact, until recently it was not unusual for nurses to give sugar water to infants at birth who were waiting for their mothers to recuperate from childbirth

Sugars enter your body and are almost instantly rushed to your brain and heart, giving these organs an immediate feeling of energy and well-being. Sugar also robs the body of calcium, thereby promoting tooth decay. And sugar creates a dependency as strong as any other addictive drug. If you stop eating sugar completely, you are likely to experience withdrawal symptoms.

The typical high-sugar American diet comes with an enormous price tag of neurosis, hypoglycemia, diabetes mellitus, cancer of the biliary tract, colorectal cancer, arthritis, arteriosclerosis, coronary insufficiency and more. The average American consumes 170 pounds of sugar annually.[18] In other words, most people eat more than their entire body weight in sugar in one year!

You may think those estimates don't include you because you don't eat a lot of candy. The fact is that most of that sugar intake—a whopping 66 percent—comes camouflaged in processed un-foods! Even with increased public awareness of the dangers of sugar, the average individual continues to consume 25 percent of all his or her calories from sugar.

You would think that it would not be difficult to eat less than 30 pounds of sugar a year—one-fourth of the entire body weight of a small- to medium-sized woman. Eating this moderate amount of sugar insures you of less illness and a strong tendency to live longer. For example, the Seventh Day Adventists eat a vegetarian diet and avoid preservatives and refined foods. It is no coincidence that they live an average of twelve years longer than the rest of the population.[19]

The death of fiber

The most severe death sentence handed to our food supply from the food industry was the death of fiber. Fiber never stood a chance—it was virtually completely wiped out. Living cancer free and maintaining a general state of good health depends upon our capacity to adequately nourish ourselves and eliminate waste. Fiber has the life-saving task of helping our bodies eliminate waste. Without proper elimination, dangerous and poisonous toxins remain inside our bodies, becoming increasingly rancid. If we cannot expel them quickly, our bodies are left with little choice but to reabsorb the poisons that our systems rejected for good reason. This toxic state, as we have already seen, is the seedbed of cancer.

The result of our fiber-poor diet is a chronically constipated society. This condition has perpetuated itself so strongly that even in medical schools they teach us that moving our bowels between once a day and once every three days is normal.

Research groups like H. S. Goldsmith (*Lancet*, 1975) and Reddy and Wynder (*Journal of the National Health Institutes*, 1975) reported that people in our modern Western culture produce small amounts of feces every twenty-four to forty-eight hours; these stools are hard, segmented, frequently painful and difficult to excrete. This is compared to people who eat primitive diets, fiber-rich in raw fruits and vegetables, who eliminate three times as much waste with soft and voluminous feces that are easy to excrete. And while Westerners defecate the remains of food eaten two days earlier, groups like the Hunza report a maximum intestinal transit time of ten hours. The danger of constipation is highly underestimated.[20]

Kian Liu and E. L. Wynder discovered that for every one hundred thousand inhabitants in the United States one hundred nine die of colon cancer, but only four of every one hundred thousand in Uganda. This is the quantitative difference between the modern high-tech diet and a fiber-rich diet.[21] Although their eating habits are very different, all live a long time and are seldom ill. The secret? They have very high-fiber diets that keep them from constipation and detoxify their bodies from dangerous, cancer-causing poisons.

English experts like J. Yuddkin from London in 1972 and later in 1974, T. L. Clave from Bristol, reported high incidence of cancer in peoples from the modern Western world because of diets rich in fats and refined foods resulting in constipation.

Later Wilkins and Hackman published similar findings in Americans.[22] Their feces contained elevated quantities of nitrogen, fat, cholesterol, biliary acids and a high concentration of carcinogenic metabolites, which are chemical wastes produced as our body metabolizes the adulterated food.

Dr. Adlercreutz, in his article "Diet, Mammary Cancer and Metabolism of the Sex Hormone," underlines the fact that Western women enjoy unrestrained consumption of animal proteins and fats, along with refined carbohydrates. This low-fiber diet not only increases their risk of colon cancer, but it also substantially increases the production of estrogens. This excessive endogenous estrogen—that normally should be eliminated through the stool—is trapped in the colon by constipation and easily reabsorbed into bloodstream concentration.

In contrast, Oriental women who eat high-fiber, unprocessed foods avoid this deadly cycle. Their hormones tend to be much more stable because of their superior diet and good detoxification. It is now commonly accepted that high-fiber diets increase expectancy for good health.

Though we have pointed the finger at harmful estrogen and estrogenic chemicals, we must note that not all estrogens are harmful. Vegetables such as the soybean, broccoli and the pomegranate offer us phytohormones or phytoestrogens, which protect us from carcinogenic mutations. Typically, diets that contain good amounts of these and other phytoestrogen-rich foods help to fight against disease. Chinese and Japanese women eat foods rich in good estrogen such as tofu, soy and miso. They seldom develop cancer, and curiously, they rarely suffer osteoporosis or any of the diseases related to low estrogen production after menopause.

Death by diet

Our generation has been fed on processed, devitalized dead foods. As a result, we have become one of the most overfed and undernourished cultures on earth. Our diet has exposed us to cancer and other degenerative diseases that might otherwise have been prevented.

Children are especially affected by our poor diet in dramatic ways. Their bodies need plenty of rich, wholesome food that they are not getting. Instead, they are growing up in today's fast-food, junk-food world. Teeth, cells, bones, muscles and vital tissue are being built from materials that are worse than inferior; in many respects they are deadly, as we have discussed.

Mental havoc. The consequences of our lack of proper nutrition don't stop with increased threats of physical disease. Eating dead, toxic food has affected our intellectual abilities as well. A serious increase in behavioral problems in children and adolescents can be directly attributed to poor nutrition.

Overaggression in youth is linked to eating refined sugars found in sweets and sodas.[23] Jails are a showcase for this behavioral problem. In one of them a dietary experiment was carried out in which fruit, fresh vegetables and water were substituted for sweets, cookies and sodas. After this healthy change of diet, aggressiveness and other behavior problems among the prisoners were reduced remarkably in just a couple of weeks![24] This simple, inexpensive experiment clearly demonstrates the relationship between behavioral problems and diet.

Vitamin and mineral deficiencies affect the biochemical balance that controls the neurotransmitters in the brain. According to researchers from Massachusetts Institute of Technology, this crucial alteration leads to learning and behavioral dysfunction.[25] This is by no means a new discovery. In 1790 (not 1970) at the Tuke's Clinic in York, England, complete wards of patients diagnosed with dementia were emptied when a regimen of nutritious foods was implemented.[26]

In the Cleveland Clinic, twenty teenagers with neurotic problems were found to have a severe thiamin deficiency.[27] After their failure to respond to treatment with conventional methods, the doctors treated them with thiamin instead. The alternative treatment produced either marked improvement or total remission of the symptoms.

Thiamin, also called vitamin B$_1$, is necessary for carbohydrate metabolism and normal neural activity. Lack of thiamin causes beriberi, a disease that can cause neurological symptoms, behavioral dysfunction, disorientation and delirium. A deficiency of vitamin B$_3$ also causes Pellagra, a disease characterized by psychiatric symptoms such as dementia as well as depression, diarrhea and skin problems. A simple dietary change is able to bring noted improvement to mental problems.

Some say that more people have died from the typical American diet that includes dead, devitalized, refined, overprocessed foods than in all the wars combined. When you take into account the cancer and heart disease deaths caused by this diet, I tend to agree with them. If you considered the diets of pins and bolts and a pulverized bus totally incredible, then think about what you're eating the next time you pick up your fork. Perhaps we're not much more sane than these poor individuals in our choices of food.

The most powerful weapon we have to use to insure and maintain health is our power of choice. Though our world has been terribly affected by modernization of food processing and even agricultural issues, we still have major choices to make when it comes to what we eat. It is up to us not to load our bodies with sugars, fats and dead foods when what we need is the kind of nutrients that bacteria and bugs crave. Choosing to eliminate even a few of the dead foods to which we are addicted could lengthen our life and increase the quality of our health immensely. The choice is ours.

What Should We Then Eat?

Sitting in front of my computer, surrounded by scores of scientific papers, health books and a head full of bright ideas, it is quite easy to chastise you and make recommendations for your healthy lifestyle. However, I do not fail to realize that walking the aisles of modern food stores confronts us all with the real, powerful and tempting allure of the food industry: convenience!

The real food is relegated to the chilly and inconvenient perimeter of most grocery stores. For every real food sold by your grocer, there are hundreds of un-food choices, which are tastier and obviously conveniently packaged for the mother-on-the-go to prepare.

I ask myself, *What would bacteria do if they entered one of our modern supermarkets?* Then I answer my own question: They would run for their lives unless the food store had an organically grown food section. Fortunately in the United States this inconvenient and more expensive organic section is becoming more and more popular. Though sacrifices must be made to pay the price and to care for these real foods, it is not as inconvenient as you might think. And in this very modern era, there is increasing demand for real foods as more people are making those choices and enjoying the benefits they bring.

Anyone who is willing to look for practical ways in which they can improve the quality of their diet will be surprised at how possible it is to do and how great the rewards will be in the quality of their life. Radical change is not always necessary, and definitely not for the first step out of the typical "dead food" American diet. Eliminating a few toxic foods and adding a few living foods will be a great start to aiding your body's built-in healing process.

The Mediterranean Diet

The "French paradox," as it is known in scientific circles as well as on the street, is the enigma that the life expectancy of the French people as compared to Americans is longer. Scientists cannot understand why, when the French eat more fat and consume more red wine than Americans, they experience less heart attacks, lower incidence of cancer, spend one-third the money on healthcare as Americans and enjoy a longer life span. Sadly, the technocrats cannot take credit for this paradox, because the longevity of the French is not a result of medical and technological advances; it is a result of ancient cultural dietary habits.

Of course not all the peoples of the Mediterranean countries eat exactly the same diet. But their rates of coronary heart disease and cancer are significantly lower, with the lowest death rates and longer life expectancy (among these Mediterranean cultures) occurring in Greece. Though their diets are similar, they differ in the amount of total fat and olive oil they consume, the types of meat they eat, wine intake, milk vs. cheese and fruits and vegetables. Here are the common denominators in the Mediterranean diet:

- High monounsaturated/saturated fat ratio (olive oil)
- Moderate alcohol consumption (red wine during meals)
- High consumption of legumes
- High consumption of whole grains
- High consumption of fruits
- High consumption of vegetables
- Low consumption of meat and meat products
- Moderate consumption of milk and dairy products

Extensive studies of traditional diets indicate that a Greek's diet consists of a high intake of fruits, vegetables (particularly wild plants), nuts and cereals (mostly in the form of sourdough bread rather than pasta); more olive oil and olives; less milk but more cheese; more fish; less meat; and moderate amounts of wine, more so than other Mediterranean countries.[28]

"Natural" supplements. Not only are their foods generally pesticide and chemically free (organically grown), the foods these Mediterranean cultures consume are loaded with natural cancer-fighting and heart-friendly agents that account for their natural health benefits. Analyses of the dietary pattern of the people of Crete show that a number of protective substances are found naturally in their diets. These include selenium, glutathione, a balanced ratio of omega-6 to omega-3 essential fatty acids, high amounts of fiber and antioxidants such as vitamins E and C, which have been shown to be associated with lower risk of cancer, including cancer of the breast.

A little wine, please. Resveratrol (found in grapes and wine and polyphenols from olive oil) is a promising anticancer agent for both hormone-dependent and hormone-independent breast cancers, and it may mitigate the growth stimulatory effect of linoleic acid in the Western-style diet.[29]

Phytochemicals found in grapes and wine, like resveratrol, have also been reported to have a variety of anti-inflammatory, anti-platelet and anticarcinogenic effects.[30]

A nutty snack. Instead of snacking on high-caloric, fat-laden, chemically rich processed junk food, Mediterranean people quiet their between-meals appetite by eating nuts. This is very smart because studies have reported that almond consumption may reduce colon cancer risk. Western dieticians, ignorant of the health benefits of nuts, have scared us away from eating them because of their high fat and caloric content. However, almonds and other nuts appear to confer important health benefits despite their high fat content.[31]

> The longevity of the French is not a result of medical and technological advances; it is a result of ancient cultural dietary habits.

Bring on the tomato sauce. Tomato sauce (not catsup), one of the main ingredients of the Mediterranean diet and the primary source of bioavailable lycopene, was associated with an even greater reduction in prostate cancer risk, especially for the more aggressive and life-threatening extraprostatic cancers. Harvard Medical School researchers reported recently in the *Journal of the National Cancer Institute* that lycopene intake, a carotenoid from tomatoes, was associated with reduced risk of prostate cancer.[32]

Cancer prevention diet. Dr. Jang from the Department of Surgical Oncology at the University of Illinois at Chicago says that the Mediterranean diet has the potential to prevent the three major stages of the development of cancer:

- Anti-initiation activity was indicated by its antioxidant and antimutagenic effects, inhibition of the hydroperoxidase function of cyclooxygenase (COX), and induction of phase II drug-metabolizing enzymes.

- Antipromotion activity was indicated by anti-inflammatory effects, inhibition of production of arachidonic acid metabolites catalyzed by either COX-1 or COX-2, and chemical carcinogen-induced neoplastic transformation of mouse embryo fibroblasts.

- Antiprogression activity was demonstrated by its ability to induce human promyelocytic leukemia (HL-60) cell differentiation.[33]

It seems to me that the results of so much research as we have just cited should have served as a strong incentive to the scientific community to test the effect of specific dietary patterns in the prevention and management of patients with cancer. Unfortunately, instead of learning from these tangible proofs, we continue to search and research for the elusive magic bullet that will cure cancer. The politics and economics of the cancer industry cloud, to say the least, the minds of our scientists.

In evaluating the complexity of the scientific data surrounding the value of diet and nutrition, some people arrive at the oddest conclusions. I received this e-mail from a skeptical medical colleague:

- Fact: Japanese eat very little fat and suffer fewer heart attacks than the British or Americans.

- Fact: On the other hand, the French eat a lot of fat and also suffer fewer heart attacks than the British or Americans.

- Conclusion: Eat what you like. It's speaking English that kills you.

This may sound comical, but too often we are willing to use less logic than this in making dietary decisions. I still wonder: *What would bacteria do?* Certainly their reaction would not be clouded by politics and money. So why don't we do as the bacteria would and eat food the way God put it on this earth, unprocessed and unadulterated.

9 Prevention Through Lifestyle

I n midlife, my friend Jack Riley traded his daily glass of bourbon, his packs of cigarettes and his junk-food diet for running shoes. He competed in runs, marathons and triathlons 644 times. His dedication first to sports and then to the cause of cancer research is a shining light.

Then, at the age of sixty-five, Jack was given three to twelve months to live. Prostate cancer that had been diagnosed five years earlier had spread. Despite the bitter news and faced with impossible odds, he entered a grueling, three-thousand-mile triathlon to raise money for cancer research.

I asked Jack why he was attempting a physical feat that most cancer-free people would not do. He told me, "I'm a competitor, and if I can do this for a good cause, then that's what life is about. I will do it as long as God gives me the physical, mental and emotional ability. I see cancer as an opposing competitor, but I don't dwell on the strengths of my competition. I choose to focus on my own performance, which is in God's hands." In a real sense, Jack was running for his life—and the lives of many others.

In Jack's mind, he wasn't merely running a race; he was running against cancer. He threw himself into the challenge. Wearing a T-shirt that announced "Cancer Doesn't Scare Me," Jack hoped to raise enough funds for cancer research during the race to beat the disease. With this hope, he set out from the beach in Tijuana, Mexico on June 5, 1998, the Worldwide Cancer Prayer Day, planning to run, bike and swim three thousand miles to the Statue of Liberty in New York City.

Jack succeeded in his race from the Pacific Ocean through thirteen cities in California and Arizona. Sadly, at New Mexico's border, the cancer-ridden body of this brave competitor gave out. He died running a race for a cancer cure. In a day when it is difficult to find heroes, Jack Riley became one of mine.

He had courage, commitment, love, integrity and focus. Whenever I feel challenged or overwhelmed, I think about my friend Jack. Though his body was fighting cancer, Jack never let it stop him from pursuing his goals. He challenged this cruel terrorist to the end with his relentless spirit and sheer determination. He once told me that cancer was an opportunity for him—an opportunity to display more courage, to allow less fear and to learn to celebrate life to the fullest doing the things he always wanted to do. In my heart, I believe that Jack was the true winner of that triathlon.

Jack's courage, determination and dedication to his sport in the face of his struggle with cancer deeply inspired my life. I wonder what would happen if each one of us displayed Jack's kind of discipline, courage and determination in our own lives in running against this formidable opponent, cancer, before it occurs? What if we determined to meet cancer's challenge to attack our own bodies with a perfect counterattack—prevention? If we displayed even a fraction of Jack's courage in our efforts to prevent the disease, I believe we would see the cancer rate (50 percent for men and 30 percent for women) dramatically reduced in a few years.

Moderate Exercise: A Major Offensive

It is not difficult to understand that the easiest and best way to beat cancer in your own body is through prevention. This offensive strategy against disease requires a lifestyle that should be pursued by everyone living in today's polluted environment. If you have had cancer or are in remission, if you have cancer now or are in a particularly high-risk group, or even if you feel it will not touch you, developing a cancer-free lifestyle is the only insurance policy available for good health. Everyone should do it.

Along with good, live nutrition and healthy detoxification, as we discussed, another key in developing a cancer-free lifestyle is ongoing, moderate exercise. Researchers concur that living a sedentary lifestyle contributes to cancer. Research from the College Study indicates that those who use up 2,000 calories or more in physical activity each week have a third less risk of getting all types of cancer as compared to sedentary individuals.[1]

Researchers believe that exercise may prevent colon and breast cancers.[2] One study found that women who exercise an average of four hours per week reduced their risk of breast cancer by 50 percent compared to that of age-matched inactive women.[3] Exercise may also help boost the immune system and even help promote such healthy habits as getting a good night's sleep.

Use it or lose it

Scientists once believed that as a species, what we stopped using we would eventually lose. If that were true we would be in serious trouble. People as a whole are more sedentary and overweight than ever before. Even the extensive research substantiating the numerous health benefits of regular exercise doesn't change this fact for many people.

According to recent reports, more than 60 percent of adult Americans do not participate in regular exercise. Perhaps more alarming is that about a quarter of them report no involvement in leisure-time physical activity at all.[4]

Fewer than a third of adults in the U.S. get the recommended amount of exercise each day, and 40 percent are almost totally sedentary. The result, as reported in December 2001 by the Surgeon General, is that obesity may soon overtake cigarette smoking in the United States as the leading cause of preventable death.[5]

Most Americans spend their days completely immobile,
either sitting in front of a computer terminal, television set, at a
desk or behind the wheel of a car. Those who live like this tend to park as closely as possible to the malls or grocery stores to save steps, and they never take the stairs.[6]

> **Obesity may soon overtake cigarette smoking in the United States as the leading cause of preventable death.**

Researchers believe that this unconscionable level of inactivity may be linked at least in part to as many as two hundred fifty thousand deaths every year in the United States—nearly a quarter of all deaths.[7]

Another study involving men who underwent two preventative medical exams several months apart showed that those
who did not improve their fitness between their first assessment
to the second had the highest mortality rates. In contrast, those
who attempted to shape up, even just a little, fared much better. Their risk was a full 44 percent lower than those who
remained unfit.[8]

These studies concur that the couch-potato lifestyle is deadly.
Research shows a close causal connection between the couch-
potato lifestyle and cancer and a raft of other deadly diseases,
including hypertension, obesity, osteoporosis, depression and
diabetes. Those who seem to be at greatest risk are women,
African Americans, low-income, less-educated populations and
the elderly.[9]

The health benefits of regular exercise are impressive. They
include preventing heart disease and stroke, improving blood
flow and cholesterol levels, reducing blood pressure and lowering
the risk of colon, prostate, endometrium and breast cancers.[10]

Walk for your life

If you are concerned that getting off the couch means that you will have to enter a triathlon, don't worry. The best exercise may not be as strenuous as you think. Brisk walking, not jogging or pumping iron, may well prove to be the perfect exercise.[11]

"Regular physical activity is probably as close to a magic bullet as we will come in modern medicine," said Dr. JoAnn Mason, chief of preventative medicine at Harvard's Brigham and Women's Hospital. Walking is one of the safest forms of exercise by far. It puts much less stress on your knees than jogging or running. If everyone in the U.S. were to walk briskly for thirty minutes a day, we could cut the incidence of many chronic diseases 30 to 40 percent, says Mason.

In my book *The Hope of Living Long and Well* I outline the benefits of the following kinds of moderate exercise. When people ask me what kind of exercise they need, I recommend that they always check first with their doctor or healthcare practitioner to see what kind of exercise is best for them. It is important that you never begin any exercise program without first seeing your doctor.

Aerobic training. Aerobic exercises are those exercises that are rhythmical and repetitious in nature, and they are good for large muscle groups. Aerobic exercises include walking, jogging, cross-country skiing, stair climbing, swimming, basketball, rowing and skating. Make sure your aerobic exercises give both your arms and legs a good workout.

Recent reports suggest that brisk walking may yield the same health benefits of strenuous exercise with far fewer injuries. The key is trading off the intensity for the duration. Benefits of brisk walking include:

- Keeping the heart in shape
- Lowering blood pressure
- Boosting the amount of good cholesterol (HDL) in the blood
- Making blood less sticky, reducing the risk of clots

- Lowering the risk of colorectal cancer by aiding elimination
- Lowering the risk of endometrial and breast cancers by reducing a woman's body fat. Body fat tends to increase the production of estrogen, which is a facilitator in the growth of some cancers.[12]

As with any therapeutic remedy, the key to reaping its benefits is to stay with it. If you walk briskly four times a week for about twenty minutes, you can expect your overall health to improve dramatically over time.

Resistance training. Training with weights can increase muscular strength and endurance in both men and women. Don't think that you are too old for weightlifting. Even if you are elderly, resistance training can still produce the most dramatic results for you.

Working with weights is especially beneficial for building bone density. "Lifting weights and other resistance training can be even more important than other forms of exercise in fighting osteoporosis and obesity," said Dr. Thomas Perls of the Harvard Medical School's Division on Aging.[13]

> Regular physical activity is probably as close to a magic bullet as we will come in modern medicine.

You don't need to pump iron with heavy barbells every day, however. Get a set with which you can do eight to fifteen repetitions without stopping. By doing eight to ten different exercises two days a week, you can realize an enormous improvement.

If you are younger than fifty, work your major muscle groups two to three days a week with weight loads that permit eight to twelve repetitions. Older patients should exercise with weight loads that allow ten to fifteen repetitions.[14]

Flexibility training. Flexibility training increases the elasticity of joints while reducing the risk of injuries. Start with a modest flexibility program two to three times a week that includes range-of-motion exercises to stretch all major muscle and tendon groups.

Establish short-term goals for yourself that are both realistic and reachable. And once again, remember that you should never begin any exercise program without first seeing your doctor or healthcare practitioner.

Some final pointers. Here are some tips that can help you move from a sedentary lifestyle to a more active one. To begin with, just move more. Becoming an active person can involve thousands of tiny little choices you make throughout your day to move around. See if these ideas can spark others for you that will help you change your paradigm of "non-movement" to simply moving more.

- Start taking the stairs instead of the elevator.
- Walk to the kitchen to get your own drink of water instead of asking someone to bring it to you.
- Walk to the mailbox instead of stopping at it when you pull into your driveway.
- Walk to the corner store to get the paper instead of having it delivered.
- Choose an outside activity like miniature golfing instead of TV.
- Take a walk along the beach.
- Take ballroom dancing lessons.
- Choose an exercise you find enjoyable—and do it.
- Plant some flowers in your front yard and spend a few evenings a week digging in the dirt.
- Walk next door to check on your neighbor instead of calling on the telephone.

These tiny decisions will act like little stones paving a road to an entirely new attitude, renewed health and energy and ultimately to a longer life. Decide today to get moving!

Meditation for Dummies

Physical exercise is vital to an overall cancer-free lifestyle. But that's only a part of the picture. Deep breathing and relaxation exercises reduce stress and help the body to maintain overall good health. In addition, if you are coping with cancer, you may discover that daily relaxation techniques can boost your overall mental and emotional outlook

During my oncological residency in Vienna I studied under some of the most brilliant and dedicated professors on earth. Once, while I was making the rounds, the mother of a patient came running to a very dedicated pediatric oncologist with a smile that her face could hardly contain. She had just received the wonderful news that her six-year-old boy was cancer free. She approached the doctor, exuding gratitude in every movement and exclaimed, "Thank God, and thank you for the miracle!"

The professor, not even stopping to acknowledge the compliment, retorted that he had not seen God during the long nights he had spent by her son's bedside; he had not seen God during the administration of the therapy; indeed, not even around the hallways had anyone seen God. The ecstatic mother stood there perplexed, along with us residents making rounds with him, not knowing what to say. He turned, and in the tone of voice he used to instruct us, admonished, "Anyone with half a brain should realize there is no God."

Apparently, the one missing a half of a brain was the good professor. Now scientists are telling us that one-half of the brain, or a portion thereof, is "wired" for religious experiences.[15]

Yet, skepticism about faith and prayer is rampant among many people. Researchers from the Department of Psychology, University of Memphis, say that from a postmodern standpoint, all trust is ultimately unfounded, in the sense that no authoritative, theoretical, empirical or practical foundation exists to ground a unified, explicit and justified framework for psychotherapeutic practice.[16] In other words, things of the mind are intangible and subjective.

These and other scientists chose to dismiss the mounting scientific evidence of emotional and spiritual power that exists. Clinical studies of mind-body interactions are paving the way for emerging paradigms in medicine.

Observations in many meditative traditions suggest a series of objective indicators of health beyond absence of disease. Several of the physical signs have been confirmed by research or are consistent with modern science. Integration of meditation with conventional therapy has enriched psychotherapy and Freudian developmental psychology.[17]

Brain-mind research at the University Hospital of Psychiatry in Zurich, Switzerland has measured the activity of different brain neuronal populations during volitionally self-initiated, altered states of consciousness that were associated with different subjective meditation states.[18]

Meditation has proven to stimulate the immune system significantly. For instance, the practice of Guolin Qigong, a combination of meditation, controlled breathing and physical movements designed to control the vital energy (qi) of the body and consequently to improve spiritual, physical and mental health, has been reported to alter immunological function. Blood levels of the stress-related hormone cortisol, a known inhibitor of type 1 cytokine production, may be lowered by short-term practice of Qigong, and there are concomitant significant increases in the IFNgamma:IL10 ratio, a definite measure of immune stimulation.[19]

Scientists evaluate prayer

In order to evaluate prayer objectively, scientists have designed studies on living entities that cannot be emotionally swayed: They have measured the impact prayer has on plants. For instance, at the Northwestern University Medical School in Highland Park, Illinois, researchers conducted a double-blind series of experiments to determine whether a process of meditation on the water (referred to as "treated") given to a controlled planting of green peas or wheat would affect their germination. They concluded that meditation upon the water (in other words, prayed for water) supplied to green peas and wheat can affect their germination rates and growth.[20]

It should not take a lot of convincing to understand that the human mind is a powerful tool that should be exploited, in the positive sense of the word, in times of need. An interesting study at the Psychology Department of the Maharishi University of Management in Fairfield, Iowa tested the effects of reading Vedic Sanskrit texts without knowledge of their meaning. The subjects experienced distinct physiological changes. Skin conductance levels significantly decreased during both reading Sanskrit and Transcendental Meditation practice, and increased slightly during reading a modern language. Alpha power and coherence were significantly higher when reading Sanskrit and during Transcendental Meditation practice, compared to reading modern languages.

Similar physiological patterns when reading Sanskrit and during practice of the Transcendental Meditation technique suggests that the state gained during Transcendental Meditation practice may be integrated with active mental processes by reading Sanskrit.[21]

There has been widespread and growing use of this approach within medical settings in the last twenty years, and many claims have been made regarding its efficacy. Mindfulness-Based Stress Reduction is a clinical program developed to facilitate adaptation to medical illness; it provides systematic training in mindfulness meditation as a self-regulatory approach to stress reduction and emotion management at the Princess Margaret Hospital and the Department of Psychiatry, University of Toronto, Ontario, Canada.[22]

Most health professionals agree that emotional and spiritual help is beneficial, yet the vast majority of nurses perceived their professional preparation in this area to be fair or poor. However, they recommend regularly or periodically four therapies:

multivitamins, massage, meditation/relaxation and pastoral/spiritual counseling.[23]

Growing bodies of clinical experience and research suggest there are major benefits for patients, physicians and alternative practitioners with the integration of meditation with conventional medical care.

A national mail survey assessing the attitudes and practices of professionals in the field of physical medicine and rehabilitation (PM&R) regarding prayer and meditation showed that although the majority of respondents endorsed prayer as a legitimate healthcare practice, there was greater belief in the benefits of meditation.[24] However, rarely will a doctor recommend prayer to a patient as a therapeutic tool, much less suggest that they both, patient and physician, get together and pray.

Interest in complementary and alternative medicine has grown dramatically over the past several years. Cancer patients are always looking for new hope, and many have turned to nontraditional means. Eighty percent of patients reported using some type of alternative therapy. Meditation and deep breathing were the two most common relaxation techniques practiced.

In light of the growing interest in alternative therapies, healthcare professionals need to be educated about the most common therapies used and hopefully use them for the benefit of their patients.[25]

So called primitive peoples of the world share a philosophy that human interaction via ceremony or ritual can affect the natural world.[26] Modern, sophisticated skeptics would consider these people half-brained, God-fearing fools. It shows that half their brain is wiser than most full-brained oncologists.

I encourage you to meditate on the wonder and the power of your mind and spirit; however, I urge you to meditate even more in the God who gave you that power and reach for His guidance and strength. If reading unintelligible Sanskrit will improve your immune system, imagine what the loving words of God will do for you. The Scriptures record the benefits of meditating on God:

I meditate on all thy works; I muse on the work of thy hands.

—Psalm 143:5, kjv

When I remember thee upon my bed, and meditate on thee in the night watches. Because thou hast been my help, therefore in the shadow of thy wings will I rejoice. My soul followeth hard after thee: thy right hand upholdeth me.

—Psalm 63:6–8, kjv

Our lifestyle does play a large part in the prevention as well as the treatment of disease. A willingness to learn how to make even the slightest lifestyle changes can result in a dramatically increased quality of life that can serve both to maintain health as well as aid the healing process.

10 Environment: Our Responsibility

A number of years ago, I was invited to an Amish community to give a lecture on alternative therapies against cancer. The more I got acquainted with this good community, the more I felt as if the hands of my watch had spun backwards and time had transported me back to seventeenth-century America. Few roads in the community were paved, people traveled by horse-drawn carriage, farmers plowed fields walking behind teams of horses or oxen, and there was no electricity, no televisions or no radios. Even the people's black attire reminded me of movies I had seen about the first immigrants from England.

Not only did these gracious folk warmly welcome me to their gentle community, but everything about their lives demonstrated to me the true meaning of love and respect they have for all of nature. The Amish are an ultraconservative Christian culture that seeks to live life according to a strict interpretation of biblical principles. All of their communal laws have been based on their interpretation of the Word of God.

From sunup to sundown, the Amish lifestyle is maintained through hard work and discipline. Food is produced from the earth and then preserved and eaten without altering its natural form more than is absolutely necessary. In many Amish communities, no water is piped in, nor do they have sewer drains, gas or any powered equipment or machinery. They really do work from

149

sunup to sundown, for that is the primary source of light for them.

As I visited with these kind people following my lecture, I asked them why they had rejected the technological advances of the twentieth century in favor of such a simple, though primitive, lifestyle. It seemed to me such a waste for people to reject the technological advances achieved by the intelligence that God has given man.

Their candid response to my question was that they are convinced that the downfall of man physically, morally and spiritually is directly related to technological progress and industrial advance. The profundity of this simple concept impressed me deeply. My respect for their discipline, sacrifice and dedication to biblical principles grew immensely with this enlarged understanding of their culture. And it challenged my own cultural beliefs.

We all know the cliché "The truth hurts." The truth doesn't actually harm us, but it does makes us uncomfortable. What argument could I propose to rebut their challenge? I realized I was in almost total agreement with their philosophy. Without a doubt, I believe the industrial and technological revolution is destroying mankind.

It is no accident that research has noted the Amish live some eight years longer than the average American. It was a memorable experience for me to live with the Amish for thirty-six hours. The night I spent in their community seemed to last an eternity. I was amazed at how difficult it was for me to be stripped of modern technology. I could not turn on a light to read. I could not listen to a stereo, answer a telephone or watch television.

Though I continued mulling over the lessons I had learned from the Amish, I couldn't wait to check into a hotel, take a hot bath and enjoy the conveniences of running water, flushing toilets and electricity. Our humanity demands the comfort and convenience that accompany modernization, even though we are aware we are leaving behind an overwhelming debt that must paid by generations to come. The debt of environmental destruction and atmospheric contamination will not be paid easily by those who live in the next generation. Left unpaid, the hope for a healthy future is bleak. But what do we do about it?

Stewards of Our Environment

We have a responsibility to take off our blinders and show genuine concern for our own children who are living in an environment so disastrous that it presents a real threat to their health. We must find a balance between enjoying the benefits of technology and being responsible for their price tag of environmental deterioration. Unfortunately, in the irresponsibility of our love for comfort, we have allowed our technological "progress" to become destructive.

God's original mandate for mankind was that they have dominion or rule over the earth, tending it as a garden to let it be the safe environment He created it to be. Have you ever wondered what the world would be like today if Adam and Eve had followed the destiny God gave to them? Creation must have been a beautiful, pristine sight for that original couple. The Bible records God's will for them:

> And God created man in His own image, in the image of God He created Him; male and female He created them. And God blessed them; and God said to them, "Be fruitful and multiply, and fill the earth, and subdue it; and rule over the fish of the sea and over the birds of the sky, and over every living thing that moves on the earth."
> —GENESIS 1:27–28

Unfortunately, since the fall of mankind, we have not only been irresponsible in cultivating relationship with God, but we have been equally irresponsible as the stewards of the environment in which He placed us. According to Scripture, God placed our environment into our stewardship as a holy trust.

From ancient times to our modern civilization, world leaders have not considered imposing preventative measures for preserving the integrity of the environment in which they lived. Rather, they waited for disaster to occur, then worked to establish ways to fix the damage already done.

New Types of "Plagues"

Most people are familiar with the plagues God visited on Pharaoh and the Egyptians because this godless leader would not let God's people go. Those were supernatural judgments that brought destruction to their environment because of man's disobedience to God. The plagues we are facing today have the same potential for destruction that those ancient plagues caused. The difference is that today's plagues are mostly a result of our irresponsible actions in caring for our environment.

Environmental diseases

Constantly increasing levels of modern environmental contamination are causing a new type of plague known simply as *environmental diseases*. These are diseases that increase to epidemic proportions as a result of environmental stimuli. They either did not exist in earlier times or were rarely seen. Some of these diseases are easy to recognize, such as cancer, cardiovascular diseases, arthritis and the explosion of respiratory diseases in large cities. Others have a more complicated diagnosis.

In general, we lump together environmental diseases that are difficult to identify under one heading: *allergies*. For example, in Wimberley, Texas, a group of ecologically challenged people has had to take extreme measures for survival, isolating themselves from the outside world. When family and friends come to visit them in their controlled environment, conversation with them can only take place by means of an intercom system.

No visitor may enter this waiting room without fulfilling a series of strict requirements. Visitors' clothes must be made from natural fibers and must not contain any dyes. Visitors themselves must not wear any kind of perfume, lotion, soap or deodorant. They cannot bring magazines or newspapers with them because of the irritant, toxic odor of ink. The list of requirements for visitors is endless.[1]

These patients do not represent some religious sect, nor is it some group of crazy environmentalist visionaries. They are simply acute sufferers of a twentieth-century disease called *multiple chemical sensitivity*. According to Delfin Garcia in the magazine *Muy interesante*, many chemical substances in the culture today can cause humans to develop a hypersensitivity even to natural elements such as water and air. Consequently, these patients who suffer from environmental disease are ambushed by contamination that comes from common elements within the home.

Don't drink the water.

Although many of us may not be this sensitive to the myriad of contaminants in the world around us, the increasing contamination of the world's water supply poses a real threat to all of us. Humanity has always used the seas as a giant natural trash can, believing that various biological cycles living in the sea absorb waste and purify the water. However, we can now prove that in water there exists a fragile natural balance generated by its chemical, physical and biological elements.

Dumping residual waters, filled with chemicals and other waste, into the sea in an uncontrolled fashion has disrupted this delicate balance and converted some coastal regions into an environment where dangerous bacteria thrive. For decades we have experienced the tragedies of the threat these bacteria create for the populace. For example, in 1973 Italian fishermen harvested contaminated mussels that produced a severe epidemic of cholera in Italy. (Please see Appendix F for more discussion of water contamination.)

Water pollution continues to be an environmental problem that plagues all of us. Linda Gillick lives in the village of Toms River, New Jersey with her twenty-year-old son Michael. Since age three Michael has suffered from a brain cancer called neuroblastoma. Michael is one of the one hundred three children from the township who are part of the nation's largest child cancer cluster.[2]

Brain and nervous system cancers and acute lymphocytic

leukemia represent the majority of cancers attacking children. Clusters of these cases are occurring in regions where drinking water has been contaminated by carcinogenic volatile organic compounds discharged by industries and municipalities into underground sources of drinking water.

Volatile organic compounds identified by the Environmental Protection Agency as potential cancer-causing agents are associated with the child cancer clusters in Toms River, New Jersey; Winona, Texas; Port St. Lucie, Florida and Woburn, Massachusetts.[3]

It is a known fact that drinking water, including bottled water, may contain contaminants such as microbes, radionuclides, disinfectants and other contaminants. The presence of contaminants does not necessarily indicate that water poses a health risk. However, many of them do cause negative effects. Fecal *Coliform* and *E. coli* are bacteria whose presence indicates that the water may be contaminated with human or animal wastes. Microbes in these wastes can cause short-term effects such as diarrhea, cramps, nausea, headaches or other symptoms. However, many other contaminants are cancerogenic.[4]

Responsible action would make our water sources a priority to safeguard and replenish. These natural resources so vital to life and health must be protected if we are to rid ourselves of life-threatening disease.

The air we breathe

Not only is water vulnerable to industrial wastes, but industry also pours tons of sulfur dioxide and other toxic substances into the air each day. We seldom think about the toxic gases in the air we breathe. Yet, cancer, pulmonary diseases, allergies and fatigue are on the rise due to these toxins. The Environmental Protection Agency's Toxic Release Inventory has reported that nearly two billion pounds of toxic chemicals are released into our air annually.[5]

In the last decade, Mexico City's government revealed that

steadily rising levels of air pollution were creating a serous health hazard. More than sixteen million tons of contaminants are being produced there each year, of which 65 percent are originated by vehicles.[6]

Pollution from automobiles. The gasoline needed to fuel the world's billions of cars every year releases many toxins into the air supply, the most dangerous of which is lead. Lead is also found in water pipes, plastics, ceramic containers and products painted with oil paints. Children are very susceptible to lead poisoning. The symptoms of lead poisoning include stomachache, constipation, vomiting, hyperactivity, diminishing IQ, aggressive behavior, attention-deficit disorder, impaired vision, impaired hearing, slow reaction time, slow growth and poor balance.

Lead poisoning is often misdiagnosed. In the last decade, the Secretary of Health and Human Services in the United States declared that lead poisoning is the most common environmental disease and socially the most devastating among small children. Any amount of lead poisoning, no matter how minute, can lead to brain lesions, neuropsychological dysfunction, behavior problems, mental retardation, kidney problems and death.

Breathing smog. Thousands of other toxic elements are released into the air supply producing a toxic soup known as smog. Smog is a product of hydrocarbon, nitrous oxide and other particles that, upon being exposed to sunlight, become toxic. Although in some countries like Japan, Germany and the United States, standards have been established that attempt to control toxic emissions, in many other developing countries, no regulations exist.

The main source of smog is the toxic emissions from motorized vehicles. A study by the University of Southern California demonstrates the damage caused by smog. Researchers performed autopsies on one hundred young auto accident victims from the Los Angeles area. They found severe smog-related damage to the lungs of all these young people.[7]

Our bodies are not designed to ingest smog particles; we have no way to expel them. Thankfully, some of these toxins are eliminated by the kidneys. But smog particles that are not eliminated often pass into the bloodstream and accumulate in fatty tissue and other cells.

Trees: Our oxygen source

Nature depends on trees to cleanse the air. This system is very effective, but it cannot keep up with the astronomical quantities of contaminants we produce. In addition, by exploiting our natural resources, we tear down this natural layer of defense. Worldwide, less than 55 percent of the forests remain intact, which has reduced the total amount of oxygen in the atmosphere. If deforestation continues at its present rate of 4 percent of the earth's surface per year, no forests will be left by the year 2035. There should be genuine global concern about deforestation because trees play a crucial role in the cleaning of our air supply.

The average American citizen consumes seven times as much commercial wood and paper as citizens in other countries. Americans throw away the equivalent of thirty million trees in newsprint per year. Recycling a 2½-foot stack of newspapers saves one 20-foot pine tree. Besides supporting measures such as enforcement of laws that protect our trees, there is a lot we can do as individuals for them.[8]

Acid rain

"Good morning," said the weatherman of a radio station in Los Angeles. "The satellite shows a possibility of 80 percent *acid* rain today; take your umbrella, and may God be with you!"

The United States releases more than seventy-four thousand tons of sulfuric dioxide into the atmosphere every day among many thousands of other impurities. These include nitrous oxide, hydrocarbons, carbon monoxide, lead and fluorocarbons that destroy the ozone layer. Rain made up of water and contaminants—especially sulfuric oxide and nitrous oxide—is dropped to the earth as acid rain.

The contaminants can also be mixed with snow or dust. The

effect of acid rain on plants, seas, lakes and rivers, not to mention humans, is incredible. It is responsible for wiping out the marine life in several lakes in Canada as well as some in Europe.[9]

Global warming

In the past few years, global warming has been blamed for everything from fires to floods and hurricanes. This ecological "greenhouse effect" is created by the massive amounts of carbon dioxide being released into our atmosphere. This causes ultraviolet light from the sun to hold heat, thus raising the earth's temperature. Through time the oceans recede and leave sandy beaches. Scientists consider that in this case sandy beaches would be enormous. Eventually fertile fields will become deserts.

"Miscellaneous" contamination

There are a host of dangerous toxins that fall into four categories:

- Synthetic organic chemicals such as benzene and many pesticides
- Natural chemical substances such as chlorine, ammonia and hydrogen fluoride
- Toxic fibers such as carcinogenic asbestos
- Toxic metals such as mercury, nickel and cadmium

Government testing is impossible against such an ocean of the millions of synthetic organic chemicals produced by industry. If a substance is tested and proven harmful, its production may be banned. But when laws are applied, they merely "Band-Aid" the gushing wound, for industry giants then seek out a Third World country in which to produce their products.

Disposal of special wastes

Special wastes are substances generated by industry, agriculture or the government that must be disposed of in a special or extraordinary way. It is estimated that in the United States of

America, one ton of toxic wastes per person is produced every year by the commercial industry.[10] But the U.S. military industry generates about one ton of toxic waste every minute, from chemical weapons to lethal radioactive materials.[11] Special wastes are extremely expensive to manage. Many countries lack the resources to adequately dispose of these dangerous materials.

Illegal uses of these wastes are hard to monitor because of their sheer quantity. For example, in May of 1971, at the Shenandoah Stables in St. Louis, approximately two thousand gallons of oil were spread on the ground to control the dust stirred up in the arena where the horses were trained. This is a common practice in this business, but oil companies are required to remove any toxic materials before selling oil to be used for these purposes.

Birds, cats and dogs in the vicinity where this oil was spread soon began to die. Of the eighty-five horses quartered at the stables for training purposes, forty-three died within a year. It was not long before the owners of the stables began to suffer headaches, chest pains and severe diarrhea. Several studies were conducted in an effort to find out what was causing this inordinate suffering and death.

Tests showed that the oil poured on the soil contained dioxin, a highly toxic contaminant. Unfortunately for the wildlife, livestock and the people living in this area, this contaminant had not been removed from the oil before it was applied to the ground.[12] This illegal and irresponsible act was only one of many such incidents like it that take place every day in the world.

Thousands of tons of toxic sediments are filtered out of industrial discharges continually. These special wastes, especially those that are radioactive, are buried deep underground in special airtight, sealed containers. Still, who can say whether or not over time such containers could leak these poisons into the soil and water.

In the United States, toxic residues are simply driven to one of over thirty thousand official storage sites. It is calculated that many toxic materials are also stored in some fifty thousand clandestine warehouses.[13] The government is aware of their existence, but they do not act to close down these warehouses because the legal waste sites cannot handle the volume of toxic materials produced.

The incidence of environmental disease in America is much higher in urban areas near stockpiles of toxic materials. The Environmental Protection Agency reported that in two hundred forty counties studied, the incidence of breast cancer was significantly higher in counties that contain nuclear facilities or radioactive waste dumps.[14] These waste sites are often located near the poor, increasing their exposure to cancer-causing agents and consequently their cancer rates.

In Mexico and many other countries, resources for storing waste are much more limited. In 1993, Mexico reported that only forty-two companies existed in the entire country for the management, treatment and disposal of special wastes. Sadly, this means that enormous quantities of these toxic materials end up in ordinary dumps.

Nuclear contamination

Radioactive particles introduced into the environment from nuclear explosions and nuclear power plants have worried physicists for decades. Communities in the United States have complained about the amount of nuclear tests performed in the deserts of Nevada and Utah since 1950.[15] For many years, evidence has existed about the dangers of exposure to the residue of such detonations. No action was undertaken by the United States government until 1984 when a federal judge in Utah ruled that ten persons had developed cancer as a result of the radiation produced by military testing.[16] (Please see Appendix G for further discussion of nuclear contamination.)

The combined exposure to environmental toxins is reflected in the ever-increasing rates of cancer. An astonishing 50 percent of all men are expected to develop cancer at some time in their lives, and 30 percent of women.[17] The burden to our bodies of increasingly compounded toxicity is one of the greatest culprits. And if there is not a radical change of governmental policies, it promises only to get worse.

Indoor pollution

When smog gets really bad in California, the elderly and those with allergies may be warned to stay inside. Yet, are these people really safe indoors? Another source of dangerous toxins is indoor pollution.

Office workers frequently suffer from unexplainable irritation of the eyes and skin. When customers and employees of a bank in Encino, California experienced headaches, nausea and vomiting, officials determined that the cause was an excessive concentration of carbon monoxide, indoor pollution that was twenty times greater than concentration accepted in smog-contaminated air![18]

It's possible that indoor pollution could become a greater health threat than smog. Allergist Dr. Alfred Zamm discovered that the air inside the typical American home contains "carbon monoxide, nitric acid and nitrogen dioxide in concentrations up to four times the maximum level accepted by federal guidelines."[19] Our homes and office buildings often lack adequate ventilation, so pure air is limited and harmful toxins can reach very high levels.

The best-known indoor polluters are asbestos, formaldehyde and lead. Asbestos is highly prized for its cost effectiveness and resistance to heat; almost all buildings have asbestos, particularly school buildings. In the U.S. about fifteen million children are exposed to it. Yet, it's been proven to cause of asbestosis, malignant mesothelioma and lung, mouth, larynx, esophagus, stomach, kidney and colon cancer.[20] Many developed countries have started to abandon the use of this material. But it's too late for the eleven million individuals who will die from cancer caused by asbestos products.

Formaldehyde is another toxin found indoors. Certain textiles, plywood, rugs and molded plastics contain formaldehyde. It is also found in deodorants, shampoos, hair conditioners, tooth paste, mouthwash, detergents and room deodorizers.

Experts calculate that we are in constant contact with some thirty-four thousand highly toxic man-made products that our body cannot metabolize or neutralize.[21] These products are found in our own homes, schools, churches, theaters, stores and offices.

We cannot turn back time, but we can get involved in making this world a better place by being good stewards of our environment.

Commitment to a Cleaner World: Part of the Cure

Though the challenge may seem overwhelming, a major component of the coming cancer cure will include a greater commitment to a less toxic planet. We must be willing to take the challenge; it has to start somewhere. I believe each one of us has a moral obligation to the health of humanity to do all that we can to reduce the earth's toxic burden.

Although the fringe fanatic groups have sometimes cast environmental causes in a bad light, this doesn't absolve us of our responsibility to promote the health of all of God's people. Some time ago, the United Nations held a World Summit in Rio de Janeiro, Brazil to begin addressing this issue.[22] Some of the principles proclaimed there, if fulfilled, would go a long ways to protecting our natural environment. They declared that:

- Countries should cooperate with a spirit of world solidarity, protecting and reestablishing the health and integrity of the world's ecosystem.

- Countries should enact effective laws relating to the environment.

- Countries should discourage or halt the relocation and transfer to other countries of substances that cause serious environmental degradation or that are considered dangerous to human health.

- National authorities should strive to promote the internationalization of environmental costs and the use of economic instruments, and those that pollute should bear the cost of contamination.

- Information should be supplied regarding disposal activities that could have substantial noxious impact on environments across borders.

Although the nations involved displayed solidarity regarding these environmental principles, the sad reality of such agreements is that few countries keep their promises. Even during this history-making meeting, the United States, China and OPEC strongly opposed any attempt to regulate toxic gas emissions, despite the overwhelming evidence that toxic gases are the major cause of acid rain, which is so detrimental to all life forms.

A breathtaking view

One of the most beautiful places on earth is located at the base of the Matterhorn Mountain, located on the border of Switzerland and Italy in the Pennine Alps. It's one of those places that make you gasp in awe when you see it. The Matterhorn is a favorite subject of painters, poets and writers, as well as a favorite resort for skiers, mountain climbers and tourists from all over the world.

When my family and I had a chance to visit the Matterhorn I didn't doubt for a moment that we would go. We took the automobile trip with some friends, but the highway ended a long way before we arrived at the famous mountain. We had to park the car and board an electric train. This seemed a major inconvenience, especially for those of us who were traveling with small children.

The citizens of that region had pledged to protect the purity of their environment, so gas- and diesel-motorized vehicles were not allowed. To travel in the area, the local residents either walked or rode bicycles, horses or electric carts. Such "inconvenience" scares away a lot of potential tourists. Nevertheless, the residents sacrifice economic benefit for their love and respect for their environment and their desire to maintain its pristine quality for their children. For the coming cancer cure to be genuine and enduring, we will have to learn from the Swiss.

We will have to treasure an unspoiled environment as one of our most precious natural resources. Doing so will take a great deal of sacrifice, but isn't restoring the health of this generation and preserving future generations worth it? As Alfred Lord Tennyson said, "Man is man, an architect of his own destiny." We alone can be the architects of the coming cancer cure.

Simple health strategies

You may think me naive to expect modern society to turn back the clock of personal convenience in favor of preserving our environment. I would respond that it is not as naive as expecting to discover the magic bullet that will eradicate cancer or expecting politicians to actually legislate policies that will promote health.

And it definitely is not naive to cry with the Old Testament prophet Hosea, through whom God declared, "My people are destroyed for lack of knowledge" (Hos. 4:6). We can change that cry to one of hope that says, "My people live because they acquire knowledge! Not only did they become aware of their health adversaries, but they were also inspired to implement practical, personal health-promoting policies that will free them of cancer and other life-threatening diseases."

Those simple health strategies would include:

- Eating food as close to the way God created it on this earth as possible.
- Supporting organically grown produce providers who not only protect your health, but also heal our earth.
- Eating as the Mediterranean cultures eat.
- Supplementing your diet with vitamins, minerals, enzymes and antioxidative cancer-fighting phytochemicals.

- Drinking lots of clean, filtered water.
- Exercising responsibly and regularly.
- Purposing to be happy, to love life.
- Loving your neighbor as you love yourself.
- Meditating not only to discipline your thoughts, but also to acknowledge the One who made it all possible.

These strategies are not overwhelmingly difficult or unreasonable, especially when the promised reward is health for us, our loved ones and our posterity. We could be the generation that turned the tide against further destruction of our God-given environment. One committed person at a time would soon become a tidal wave of public opinion, resulting in decisive efforts to become the stewards of our earth that God ordained us to be.

Section IV

Embracing
the Cure

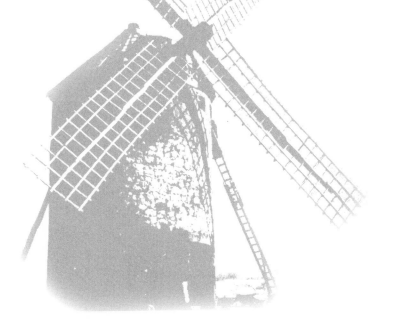

11 Weighing in With Alternative Medicine

A recent study reported in the prestigious *Journal of the American Medical Association* (JAMA) threw the orthodox medical establishment into a tailspin. This study announced that nearly twice as many individuals were seeking "alternative" healthcare at their own expense rather than conventional medical care.[1]

In 1997, Americans made 627 million visits to practitioners of alternative medicine and spent $27 billion of their own money to pay for alternative therapies. In contrast, they made only 386 million visits to their family doctor. Harvard Medical School estimates that one out of every two persons in the United States between the ages of thirty-five and forty-nine years used at least one alternative therapy in 1997.[2]

Alternative medicine is growing at an astonishing rate. Between 1991 and 1997 the use of herbal medicines in the United States grew by 380 percent and the use of vitamin therapy by 130 percent.[3]

Alternative approaches to cancer treatment are gaining greater acceptance throughout the medical community as well. Much of the reason has been the perceived failure of traditional approaches, coupled with widely heralded successes in alternative

167

methods. Only a few years ago anyone practicing alternative medicine was regarded as a quack. More recently, however, we have been elevated to alternative doctor status.

The Western Hemisphere is not alone in experiencing this strong trend toward alternative therapies. In Australia, 57 percent of the population now use some form of alternative medicine. In Germany, 46 percent have jumped on the bandwagon. In France, 49 percent are looking to alternative treatments.[4]

Researchers at Beth Israel Deaconess Medical Center and the Harvard Medical School in Boston, Massachusetts conducted a telephone survey of more than fifteen hundred adults in 1991, and then surveyed an even larger group in 1997. During this six-year period, there was a 47.3 percent popular swing to alternative medical practitioners. In 1991, 427 million adult individuals used alternative medicine; in 1997, the figure leaped to 629 million.[5] The use of herbal medicines increased by 380 percent, and megavitamin use rose 130 percent.[6]

Why Choose Alternative Medicine?

Surveyors reported that 58 percent of those surveyed sought out alternative medicines or therapies to prevent future illness or to maintain health and vitality. The remaining 42 percent used nonconventional therapies to combat existing illnesses, usually chronic conditions such as headaches, back problems, anxiety or depression.[7]

Dr. Wayne Jonas of the Office of Alternative Medicine at the National Institutes of Health in Bethesda, Maryland said he believes the increasing popularity of alternative treatments "reflects changing needs and values in modern society in general." Those changing values include an increasing skepticism toward traditional medicine, widening public access to health information and increased interest in spiritual matters.[8]

Those who use alternative treatments appear to like them well enough to stay with them, which also accounts for their growth. Some responders reported using alternative treatments for many years. Of those who tried alternative treatments, 50 percent were still using them eleven to twenty years later.[9]

The use of alternative treatments could not be classified by gender, ethnicity, level of education or whether one lived in urban or country areas. However, youth did prove to be a factor in choosing alternatives, with all age groups increasing steadily over the six-year span.[10]

The study dispels two popular notions espoused by the orthodox medical community. The first one is that alternative medical treatments are merely a passing fad; the second, they are used by only one segment of the population, according to Ronald Kessier, Harvard Medical School professor of healthcare policy, who helped to author the study.[11]

Other studies show that conventional medicine continues to be preferred in the treatment of emergencies and trauma, while alternatives excel in the treatment of chronic disease.[12]

This news sent the orthodox medical community scrambling for answers. Once allegiance to doctors was completely unquestioned. So, why are patients leaving in droves? What differences did patients see between orthodox medicine and alternative treatments? Hans Larsen suggests the following as some reasons people are choosing alternative medicine:

- Conventional medicine focuses on relief of symptoms, rarely investigating causes or methods of prevention. Alternative medicine tends to frown upon methods that mask symptoms and are much more committed to prevention.

- Conventional medicine is organ specific; hence it produces cardiologists, neurologists and so forth. Alternative medicine uses a holistic approach, seeing each person as a unique individual.

- Conventional medicine believes in the aggressive intervention to treat disease and seeks magic bullets and quick fixes. Alternative treatments prefer gentle, long-term support that facilitate the body's own healing powers.

- Conventional medicine expects a certain level of passivity from patients. Alternative medicine prefers and often requires the patient to take a highly active role in both prevention and treatment.

- Conventional medicine has traditionally resisted natural remedies, even long after their efficacy has been scientifically proven.[13]

Most alternative medicine practitioners embrace new remedies and can often point to years of safe use. For example, ginkgo biloba is now the most prescribed drug in Germany; it has been found effective in the prevention and treatment of Alzheimer's disease.[14] Also in Germany, the herb saw palmetto is prescribed in 90 percent of all cases of enlarged prostate. In the United States, three hundred thousand prostate operations are performed each year to solve the same problem.[15]

The practice of conventional medicine is intimately tied to the entire medico-pharmaceutical-industrial complex. While the first priority of most conventional physicians is healing the patient, the first priority of the medico-pharmaceutical-industrial complex is to make a profit. Many physicians find it increasingly difficult to operate within a system that subjects them to pharmaceutical salesmen, its rule books, its fear of malpractice suits, endless paperwork to satisfy bureaucrats and insurance companies and its time pressures. Alternative practitioners tend to operate free of such constraints, allowing them time to give patients the undivided attention they seek.

As we saw earlier, a major source of funding for medical research comes from pharmaceutical companies, which are reluctant to support lifestyle modifications, vitamins and other remedies that cannot be patented.[16]

With so many patients either bailing out or adding alternatives to their personal health arsenals, the conventional medical community is finding alternative medicine increasingly difficult to ignore.

The Medical Community's Response

As with any large community, you might expect a variety of different responses in the medical community to the present-day trend toward alternative medicine. There are those who are frustrated with the trend and attempt to disprove it; those who are becoming convinced that its methods are valid; and opportunists whose motivation is less than noble.

The frustrated

The frustrated continue to spend time, energy and money doing research to disprove the value of alternative methods. In an editorial in the *New England Journal of Medicine* (NEJM), editors Dr. Marcia Angell and Dr. Jerome Kassirer railed against the move to alternative medicine, blasting the industry as unscientific. "It is time for the scientific community to stop giving alternative medicine a free ride. There cannot be two kinds of medicine—conventional and alternative. There is only medicine that has been adequately tested and medicine that has not, medicine that works and medicine that may or may not work."[17]

Dr. Angell's tone of speech seemed to typify the enormous arrogance and condescension that has fueled much of the problem. She said that most consumers of alternative medicine "assume it's better because it feels better and is easier to understand." According to Angell, "many members of the public seek the more attentive, individualized care of an alternative medical practitioner, may be angry at the medical establishment and don't understand science."

Her negativity didn't stop with patients, however. Alternative doctors also lacked the ability to make sound, critical judgments as well. She said, "The long-term damage is the abandonment of critical thinking, something that will spread throughout society." She said that there has not been a widespread reaction from the medical community because, in part, doctors are not scientists and can be drawn to alternative medicine. Angell also described managers of healthcare as overly responsive to consumer demand. "HMOs are afraid, in the face of such a powerful consumer movement, to say that the emperor has no clothes. What you're up against when you pit science vs. alternative medicine is the power of the testimonial in the media. That is the toughest hurdle."[18]

Wayne B. Jonas, M.D. of *JAMA* writes, "Historically, orthodox medicine fights these practices vigorously by denouncing and attacking them, restricting access to them, labeling them as antiscientific and quackery, and imposing penalties for practicing them. When these therapies persist and even rise in popularity despite this, mainstream medicine then turns more friendly, examining them, identifying similarities they have with orthodox, and incorporating or 'integrating' them into the routine practice of medicine."[19]

The convinced

In the field of cancer, the convinced are other oncologists who are so disappointed by the poor results of traditional medicine and traditional cancer research that they have started treating their patients with a different approach. Less aggressive orthodox oncologists are quietly recommending adjuvant alternatives to patients and even encouraging them to seek alternatives in other countries.

In March 2001, I found myself in the halls of the Department of Biochemistry in London's Imperial College looking for the office of Dr. Mahendra Deonaraian and Dr. A. A. Epenetos. I had made contact with them because I found articles published about a revolutionary approach they had developed to treat cancer. It was called Antibody-Directed Enzyme Pro-Drug Therapy (ADEPT); it is also known as Antibody-Guided Enzyme Nitrile Therapy (AGENT). A particular advantage of the ADEPT approach is that it may allow the use of extremely potent agents that are too toxic to be readily used in conventional chemotherapy, delivering them directly to the malignant cells. This therapy could potentially kill cancer cells and leave the healthy tissue unharmed.[20]

Usually scientists of this caliber do not want to "waste time" with physicians like myself who use alternative therapies; nevertheless, they had an interest in what I was doing. Interestingly enough, the catalyst to our meeting was the discussion of a poisonous compound. These doctors were doing experiments with cyanide in the treatment of cancer. At our hospital, Oasis of Hope, we had been using cyanide, which is the active ingredient in Laetrile, for decades in tens of thousands of cancer patients.

Dr. Deonaraian greeted me with a handshake, and a few minutes into our conversation he said, "Dr. Contreras, we have demonstrated that this system [ADEPT] is able to specifically kill tumor cells by cyanide intoxication." The development of this treatment had been very successful in animals, and cautiously, they were setting the stage for a human study. This is a project that our Oasis of Hope research team will follow and cooperate with in any way possible. We are planning to take advantage of the research of these doctors to improve the delivery of Laetrile to the malignant cell.

When we left the meeting, I was filled with gratitude that other researchers finally vindicated the treatment my father had pioneered for cancer and that caused him so much ostracism and persecution from the medical community. Now, scientists from the medical "establishment" are telling the world that cyanide (the basis of Laetrile therapy) could be one of the best anti-tumor agents nature has to offer.

My feeling of gratitude was accompanied by sadness as well, because the medical establishment will take the credit, undeserved without question, for this "scientific discovery" of a treatment for which they criticized my father so vehemently. Still, I comfort myself with the thought that because of their affirmation of the treatment, many more patients will have access to these types of effective cancer therapies soon.

Today, the overwhelming effort is toward attempts at integrating alternative practices into the mainstream. Sixty percent of medical schools have begun to teach about alternative medicine practices.[21] Hospitals are creating complementary and integrated medicine programs.

In the past, orthodox medicine has benefited from the integration of alternative methods and treatments by abandoning ineffective treatments like bloodletting, adopting new drugs and developing more rigorous scientific methods.[22]

The opportunists

Last year, *New York Times* health columnist Jane Brody wrote, "Alternative medicine is clearly the largest growth industry in healthcare today."[23]

Don't think that the financial potential of this explosion of growth has gone unnoticed. Many doctors are integrating alternatives because they have no other choice. Patients are demanding more effective and less aggressive treatment, and the hard-core orthodox therapists are losing clientele.

For example, some hospitals in America have opened the door to chiropractic doctors and acupuncturists despite the fact that medical faculty is opposed to their treatments. They are doing so for the sole reason of attracting patients who are willing to travel out of the country seeking these services.

Recently, in response to demand and dollars and to the deep chagrin of doctors, Oxford Health Plans, Inc. of Norwalk, Connecticut, a health-maintenance organization with projected annualized revenue of about $3 billion, announced it would provide a network for alternative medical therapies as natural-remedy or "naturopathic" medicine and Chinese herbology. The big HMO plan is establishing a network of one thousand holistic providers to mirror its existing network of thirty-three thousand traditional doctors. The providers are to be credentialed much as doctors to practice in New York, Connecticut and New Jersey.[24]

Other health suppliers are offering expanded benefits packages that include services of alternative practitioners.[25]

The disillusioned

When a person turns to a doctor for help, he gives that physician his trust. Society, until recently, had accepted this norm, trusting in the integrity of the medical professional. Now, the situation is changing. Orthodox physicians are losing the public's trust, and this trend worries them.

Among the ranks of orthodox physicians is a growing number who are openly questioning the integrity of the medical community that they serve. Dr. Philip Caper, an internist and medical policy analyst at Dartmouth Medical School, concludes that the whole medical establishment leaves much to be desired: "I can't imagine a system more dysfunctional than the one we have now—more expensive, not doing the job, with more waste."[26]

Confirming this statement, the General Accounting Office (GAO) estimates that at least $200 billion U.S. are thrown away each year on overpriced, useless, even harmful treatments and on bloated bureaucracy. Every ten years, a group of private researchers for the Rand Company in Santa Monica, California takes a census of the medical practices in the United States. It reported that at least 20 percent of the procedures and treatments offered to patients are not only unnecessary, but life threatening.[27]

Annually, between twenty and twenty-five million surgical procedures are carried out among all the specialties, excluding plastic surgery. This study determined that between 15 percent and 29 percent were unnecessary. For example, 27 percent of the women who had hysterectomies, the second most common surgery, didn't need the operation. This means that between three and six million patients are submitted to surgical risk due to an improper diagnosis or for lucrative reasons.[28]

We can be grateful the anesthesiologists and intensive care specialists have managed to reduce the surgical and post-surgical death rate to 1.33 percent. This low risk still will not help the over sixty thousand patients annually who have paid with their lives for an operation they didn't need.

One of the chief tenets of the medical profession simply states, "Do no harm." Yet, the harm caused by doctors is staggering. Adverse reactions to medications recommended by physicians account for 659,000 patients hospitalized each year and sixteen thousand automobile accidents. Over sixty-one thousand people suffer the symptoms of Parkinson's disease induced by pharmaceuticals, but the tragedy of our inefficiency is shamefully exposed by the fact that each year 176,000 people die of iatrogenic (caused by doctors) diseases.[29]

The popularity of alternative medicine in this century is driven by the perception that conventional treatments are too harsh to use for chronic and non-life-threatening disease.[30]

According to Wayne B. Jonas, M.D. of JAMA, "Conventional medicine can learn from alternative medicine how to 'gentle' its approach by focusing on the patient's inherent capacity for self-healing."[31]

The High Cost of Healthcare

Skyrocketing costs of conventional medicine also are driving the search for alternatives. Healthcare costs are predicted to double over the next ten years, and who can afford these costs today?[32] In spite of deficient medical attention, hospitals charge exorbitant amounts for their services. On the TV program *PrimeTime Live* on January 12, 1995, Diane Sawyer reported that an accident victim was transported to the hospital by helicopter and spent only five hours there before expiring. His relatives were forced to pay more than $94,000 in hospital expenses and more than $10,000 for doctors' honorariums.[33] There was no doubt that the boy was treated with the sincere desire to save his life, but $104,000 for just five hours of treatment?

If low-cost interventions such as lifestyle changes, diet, supplement therapy and behavioral medicine can be delivered as substitutes for high-cost drugs and technological interventions, true cost reductions, better health and fewer deaths might occur.[34]

Response to Criticism

Recently the government created the Office for Alternative Therapies to monitor the activities of alternative practitioners. Dr. Casseleth, advisor to the Office for Alternative Therapies, summarizes their main objections to alternative medicine as follows: "While it is well to keep an open mind, it is wise to keep one's eyes open also. Many alternative therapies are not risky, except to our pocketbooks, but some can be dangerous. Do not substitute an alternative therapy for treatment already accepted."

The following are criticisms levied against alternative medicine by Dr. Casseleth to which I have responded:

Criticism: They (alternative practitioners) promise miraculous healing and offer false hope.

I agree that someone who says they are able to cure every disease has a God complex and is dangerous. Yet, supporters of orthodox medicine fail in this regard when they offer no hope and prohibit alternative treatments for conditions for which they have no viable solution. They assert that if orthodox medicine has not found a solution, there is none.

A false hope is one that has neither scientific basis nor proven results. Most alternative therapies have both. Does orthodox medicine possess a true hope? Do they have scientifically proven treatments? Many times the answer is *no*. How many times do they tell their patient: *Go home and settle your affairs because you are going to die in a few months. Don't waste money on alternative therapies.* In that statement, they destroy hope.

Criticism: Alternative treatments involve secret procedures or ingredients.

I believe that creative methodology that helps the sick should be shared. Yet, this criticism of secrecy seems very strange to me since the foundation of modern orthodox medicine is cemented with patents that protect the secrecy of drugs. Why, then, when a medical "quack" (as they regard us) discovers a method that guarantees longevity, do they censor us for being secretive?

Criticism: Alternative therapies aren't allowed to reach the public because of a conspiracy.

I counter Casseleth's cries of conspiracy with a question. How would you define the medical establishment that protects its market and investments by criticizing alternative therapies and abusing laws and rules to suppress the possibility of those therapies to survive? I call it conspiracy. You call it simply *establishment*.

Criticism: Alternative treatments involve exorbitant cost.

On the issue of cost Dr. Casseleth really failed getting the facts. No one disputes that alternative treatments are much less expensive than conventional ones. I have already mentioned that 82 percent of the patients who consulted the so-called "quacks" were satisfied with the treatment received. Who do we want to satisfy, the patients or the establishment? The cost of orthodox oncological treatments is truly exorbitant.

Criticism: Alternative therapies report exaggerated positive results backed *only* by anecdotal case histories.

In comparison to orthodox therapies for chronic degenerative diseases, the results of alternative therapies are unbelievably superior. Yet, even though they are backed by a multitude of studies, as we saw in the case of breast cancer, these studies are omitted or ignored by the orthodox medical establishment.

Criticism: Alternative therapists invite us to abandon or delay proven medical treatment.

Time and time again it has been confirmed that the conventional medical treatments are not only ineffective but also dangerous. The vast majority of patients with cancer live longer and better without the orthodox treatments. Can it be that the basis for this criticism is that alternative therapies pose a serious threat to the medical establishment that stands to lose a patient who is swayed toward alternative treatments?

Though people like Dr. Casseleth may criticize alternative doctors and treatments, the fact is that more and more doctors are becoming interested in alternative therapies. Associations like the American College of Advanced Medicine (ACAM) and others are quickly climbing on board. Hundreds of doctors are recommending or using alternative therapies in their offices. Many are satisfied with the results and are going to continue prescribing them.

I Seek Only Solutions

I have been criticized by *conventional* doctors for using alternative techniques and by *alternative* doctors for using conventional treatments like surgery and chemotherapy for the healing of my cancer patients. I do not ascribe to a system of acceptable medical treatments, either conventional or alternative. I seek only solutions for the welfare of my patients.

One of my most famous patients is Donald Factor, the son of cosmetic mogul Max Factor. When Donald came to us with advanced lung cancer that had spread to his liver, I honestly wondered if he stood a chance of surviving it. Because of the critical state of his condition, we used a Hickman catheter, an unorthodox chemotherapy treatment in which we feed medications directly into the liver. Surprisingly, he responded amazingly well, and today he continues to be cancer free, sixteen years after he was originally diagnosed. The combination of conventional and alternative therapies resulted in saving the

> I seek only solutions for the welfare of my patients.

life of this terminally ill patient.

At the Oasis of Hope Hospital, we are committed to using a proven eclectic combination of both alternative and conventional treatment strategies based solely upon our two foundational treatment pillars: Do no harm, and love your patient as you love yourself.

> **Do no harm.** We never treat a disease; we treat only patients. We approach each patient as an individual with his or her own set of needs, concerns, opinions and emotional responses. We offer only therapies that can help the patient—the whole person—without sacrificing his or her quality of life.
>
> **Love your patient as you love yourself.** If I cannot apply a particular cancer treatment to someone I love—my mother, my wife or my daughter—I cannot consider giving the treatment to anyone.

Whether physicians choose alternative therapies, conventional treatments or a combination of both approaches, my deepest desire is that as doctors we might open our eyes to all of the possibilities that promise hope for healing and a greater quality of life for our patients. An important dimension to quality of life involves spiritual issues to which we must be reconciled. As we conclude, I want to address some of these issues in a way that has been helpful to me as well as to my patients.

12 Faith for the Coming Cancer Cure

Throughout this book I have given you an overview, according to this oncologist's perspective, of the coming cancer cure. Surely you can agree with me that there is a great deal of hope on the horizon, in spite of the concerns we have discussed. I am very optimistic about the recent breakthroughs in technology as well as the new paradigm that is in place in the medical community for studying and treating the disease.

I am convinced that during these next few decades, the medical community will initiate a wonderful synergy between the molecular understanding of the cause of cancer, with its forthcoming therapies, and conventional and alternative treatments that successfully manage the disease and strongly diminish its life-threatening status.

Since 1971 when President Nixon called our nation to war against cancer, Americans have become increasingly more aware of our struggle against it. As we have discussed, a great deal of money and effort continues to promote our war against cancer on a national level. And though many of these funds have gotten muddled in a web of unproductive priorities with disappointing results, to say the efforts and expense have been wasted would be a wrong and harsh judgment.

With our increased potential for outright cancer cures and a new awareness of our ability to prevent the disease, I believe we will reverse the last century's statistical data that shows a continual rise in the rate of cancer incidences. And I believe the general population will embrace lifestyle changes as never before to assure the future prevention of cancer, not only for themselves and their children, but also for generations to come. This is the most hopeful truth about the coming cancer cure— that *cancer is essentially a preventable disease*. And even though the medical industry and cancer research bastions of power have been slow to keep pace with this reality, the masses are hearing the message and responding.

As we attack this disease in a comprehensive way, each of us taking responsibility for a cleaner environment, insisting on the pursuit of genuine cancer research along with an openness to implement alternative therapies and lifestyle changes, we will achieve our goal—the coming cancer cure.

Having concluded that there are wonderful reasons to live in hope of conquering cancer, we must still deal with the harsh realities of the present where cancer is violating humanity. For those who suffer this grief, I want to address some of your agonizing questions and offer viable solutions that have helped many of my patients. To do that we have to open our minds to the spiritual dimension of life.

Facing Incomprehensible Outcomes

I had just come back from a medical meeting where I had presented Fernando's case to a group of doctors. His amazing recovery, which we attributed in part to the practical application of ozone therapy, had created much controversy, heated debate and deep interest in the medical community regarding the treatment.

Those doctors present viewed and reviewed the CT scans. The initial x-rays showed a liver almost completely invaded by tumors the size of tennis balls. The last scan depicted a clean, tumor-free, brand-new liver. Then I discussed with them the treatment we had given him. I acknowledged to this group of doctors that even though I consider our medical aptitudes to be excellent, I attributed Fernando's recovery to a miracle from God. To this day, this is what I truly believe.

Later that week, as I was preparing to begin a new and exciting day in my practice, I looked up to see my secretary coming into my office. Immediately I recognized from her body language and facial expression that she was bringing bad news. Nothing could have prepared me for what I was about to hear.

She said, "Dr. Contreras, Fernando was killed last night in a car accident."

I was stunned. Our star ozone therapy patient who had been cured from a terminal condition, I believed, by a miracle of God, was dead? From an accident? It made no sense. *God*, I wondered, *what were You thinking?*

Fernando was virtually dead when he began our therapy. Though the effects of the therapy were nothing like the tortures of chemotherapy, he had suffered patiently and quietly the installation of a central line catheter that would enable us to perform dialysis-like procedures. These procedures were not pleasant. He was always cheerful and optimistic as he submitted to treatments and extreme changes in his diet as well as medications and supplements. Was it all for nothing?

I don't think I can describe my puzzlement, disappointment and frustration. In unexplainable, tragic times such as this, even the most deeply founded faith can be shaken. And when those around us try to explain with statements like, "God knows what He's doing," it irritates our souls and minds. At such times, in spite of the biblical authority in which we believe, out of our pain we find ourselves questioning, *Is God really there?* For those of us needing answers, God can seem far off and even angry, like the ancient and arbitrary gods of Hellenistic Greece.

Science Points to a God Who Cares

Who is to blame? Before Newton's law of causality, our ancestors believed that God was the reason for everything that happened; He was the One to blame. Then when Darwin came along and proposed that even the origins of life didn't find their source in God, faith came into question.

Now, even science in a large part is reduced to believing in a Creator. New technological advances reveal to us that we had a definite beginning. Reductionism about the function of living things and live entities has brought many scientists to the conclusion that living organisms are too complex to have simply happened by chance. Even the most reticent of agnostics seem to be coming to terms with the fact that there must be a higher purpose to this life on earth.

Albert Einstein, one of history's greatest scientific minds and an agnostic, finally acquiesced to the fact that chance—scientifically, mathematically, chronologically—did not and could not have produced the wonderful events that brought about life and the environment as we enjoy it. His scientific genius was confronted with a God he had to acknowledge reluctantly, but did not believe to be a benevolent Creator. Rather, He existed only as superior being who remained aloof and uninvolved in the daily chores of life.

Einstein believed that God could not be personal. Otherwise, how could He allow bad things to happen? He said:

> I cannot conceive of a personal God who would directly influence the actions of individuals...My religiosity consists in a humble admiration of the infinitely superior spirit that reveals itself in the little that we...can comprehend of reality. I believe in Spinoza's God who reveals himself in the harmony of all that exists, but not in a God who concerns himself with the fate and actions of human beings.[1]

Scientist Gerald Schroeder also concluded there had to be a God because, he said:

> The lottery of individual random mutations at the molecular genetic level cannot be its only driving force. A simple calculation can show that the likelihood of producing any

particular sonnet of Shakespeare by random typing is about one chance in 10 to the 690th power. So the statistical improbability of pure chance yielding even the simplest forms of life has made a mockery of the theory that random choice alone gave us the biosphere we see.[2]

While scientific advances for a while were anti-God, new discoveries are becoming pro-God. But as Arthur Peacocke put it, "More and more people are believing but not belonging."[3] Many modern scientists are now convinced that there is a God, but they do not believe that He is personally interested or involved in our lives.

Honestly addressing spiritual realities that involve a larger picture of life and purpose—God and His creation and good vs. evil—is necessary if we are to resolve the more difficult questions of life and death. Though I do not claim to be either the brightest of scientists or an enlightened theologian, I would like to offer you a practical perspective that will give you some guidance in how to cope with this controversial relationship between God and His children.

Whether we accept God as a person or not, whether we like Him or not, and even if we do not seek to know Him, relationship with our Creator is unavoidable. By virtue of having been created, as science reluctantly acknowledges, that relationship was established. Our choice is limited to using our energies to discover and strengthen a cordial relationship with God or to settle for a non-participatory or even belligerent relationship with Him. It is a scientific impossibility to ignore Him completely; His presence is seen in all His handiwork.

We live in one of the most exciting eras in the history of the universe. Scientific advances are providing us with resources to enjoy life more than ever—and not only in the material realm. New scientific evidence points toward a creation by design that has a purpose larger than the design. It even indicates that the Creator behind the design must be an entity that is emotionally attached to all events in the universe. These conclusions confirm the existence of an omniscient, omnipotent, omnipresent and caring God.

Scientist Gerald L. Schroeder concluded, "What appear to be diametrically opposed biblical and scientific descriptions of the creation of the universe, of the start of life on earth and of our human origins are actually identical realities but viewed from vastly different perspectives."[4]

It is ironic that the study of science that once caused a "debunking" of belief in a God is now so awed by creation that scientists themselves acknowledge His existence. Albert Einstein's studies led him to conclude that "the harmony of natural law...reveals an intelligence of such superiority that, compared with it, all the systematic thinking and acting of human beings is an utterly insignificant reflection."[5] And only in recent history have we begun to appreciate the complexities of the atom, of DNA and the symmetry and harmony of nature's laws.

Some scientists have even attributed this Creator God with clearly evidenced purpose, which, though He is transcendent, establishes His Personhood. Prominent scientists from Fred Hoyle to Heinz Pagels (though agnostics themselves) have written of clearly evidenced purpose or intention to bring about intelligent life in the universe. Purpose is perhaps the most important attribute of personhood, and the fact that the grand designer of the universe holds this attribute suggests that He possesses personhood.[6]

These scientists concluded, "Such a God has not needs—and yet has desires. He had not need to create the universe or us in order to sustain His existence. But it pleased Him to do so. Thus our very existence is evidence for a personal God, a God who has desires, as opposed to an impersonal force."[7]

Arthur Peacocke even suggests that God suffers with us because of who He is: "When faced with this ubiquity of pain, suffering and death in the evolution of the living world, we were impelled to infer that God, to be anything like the God who is love in Christian belief, must be understood to be suffering in the creative processes of the world. Creation is costly to God.

God is creating the world from within, and, the world being 'in' God, God experiences its sufferings directly as God's own and not from the outside."[8]

Even science concurs that there is a God who cares about our suffering as individuals He created. And if we accept the authority of the Bible as the Word of God, we find recorded there many statements regarding God's love for mankind and His desire to heal and restore our relationship with Him, which includes the healing of our bodies.

The Spiritual Dimension

Science does not, by any stretch of the imagination, explain all that is going on in this world. The deepest questions within us cannot be answered by science. For answers to the deepest issues governing sickness and health, we must open our minds to embrace a spiritual dimension of life.

The origin of disease

To answer the question of who is to blame for disease and suffering, creationists turn to the Word of God. We believe there was a time when perfect balance existed between the Creator and creation, a time of perfect health with no sickness. Adam and Eve enjoyed the cleanest, most unpolluted environment ever in Eden. Disease and death did not threaten their lives or their environment. As long as those pristine conditions existed, disease could not enter. It is not difficult to draw the conclusion that humans were designed by the Creator to live forever.

What happened? In my opinion, in the instant that first couple disobeyed the command of God to them, eating of the forbidden fruit (Gen. 2:17; 3:6), the perfect balance between Creator and creation was lost—it was broken by sin. At that moment a dramatic paradigm shift in their relationship to God occurred—the pathway to death was opened in both the physical and spiritual worlds. God's warning to Adam and Eve now haunts the human race: "But from the tree of the knowledge of good and evil you shall not eat, for in the day that you eat from it you shall surely die" (Gen. 2:17).

Now, as involuntary "sons of Adam," instead of being born to live forever, we are born, we grow, we reproduce ourselves, and then we die. Sin disrupted the perfect balance between God and man and opened the door for illness to rush in. The Bible clearly teaches that the wages of sin is death, and death is directly linked to the gradual loss of health (sickness).

For those who think this biblical concept of the "original" cause of death seems harsh, it may be interesting to note that it is not unique to the Judeo-Christian heritage. Many world religions incorporate spiritual rituals for healing that require repentance and asking of forgiveness for any transgressions that may have brought the disease upon them. This commonality of religious thought suggests that all of humanity have a deep sense that sickness is unnatural; it's not the way God intended life to be.

While some may say that all disease is the consequence of personal sin, it seems to me that is obviously not the case. For example, if you unknowingly eat contaminated food, most likely you will visit the bathroom many times during the night

> ## Sickness is unnatural; it's not the way God intended life to be.

because the balance of nature was violated. It would be hard to conclude that the cause of that episode of illness was personal sin.

Jesus clearly taught His disciples that disease is not always due to sin. Walking past a blind man on one occasion, Jesus' followers asked Him, "Who sinned, this man or his parents, that he should be born blind?" Jesus responded, "It was neither that this man sinned, nor his parents; but it was in order that the works of God might be displayed in him" (John 9:2–3). Jesus did not blame this man for his blindness. His answer indicated simply that there was a higher purpose for this man's condition. Here we glimpse the sovereignty of God at work as well for the ultimate good of mankind.

The power of prayer

In 1997, the executive vice president of the Oasis of Hope Hospital, Daniel Kennedy, approached me with a vision about starting a day of prayer for the healing of people who have cancer. He told me that he had seen the positive impact we were having on cancer patients but that we were only treating about six hundred patients per year. He had a burden for expanding our positive impact on cancer patients in every nation, and that is when it came to him. Though the one-hundred-bed hospital could not treat the tens of millions of people with cancer, we could apply a therapy to every single cancer patient. The therapy he was talking about was one that my father and I had been prescribing for our entire careers. It is the only therapy that I know of that is effective, nontoxic and free. It was the powerful healing agent *prayer*.

I gave my support to the vision, and on June 5, 1998, we founded the Worldwide Cancer Prayer Day with Dr. Robert A. Schuller from the Crystal Cathedral. Since then, we have gained the support of people and ministries in one hundred sixty countries as we get together each year in June to pray.

I do believe that God heals people, and I believe that He can prevent the occurrence of cancer in people, but I have a very special prayer that I lift up every year. I pray, "God, please grant wisdom to the doctors and scientists and help them find the cure for cancer." I believe that God will answer this prayer, and though the glory for the cure for cancer may be given to a researcher in some university, I know that it will be God who will give the enlightenment to that researcher.

Some remarkable things have happened since the first Worldwide Cancer Prayer Day in 1998. I personally have come across better therapies and am getting much better results with my patients. I thank God for that. But as amazing as it might seem, something changed in the mortality rate statistics that the American Cancer Society projected for the year 1999. Since the early 1970s, each year the projected deaths for all cancer sights increased dramatically until an all-time high in 1998 of 563,000. But in 1999, for the first time in three decades, the American Cancer Society projected a slight decrease in deaths from cancer. The explanation was that better treatment options were helping more people stay alive. Those who do not accept God's involvement in our lives would probably not see the significance, but it caught my attention. For thirty years, the mortality rate of cancer increased until one day in 1998 when people of many nations prayed to God for help—and the next year, there was a slight decrease in the death rate.

It is a wonderful experience that we have now as we receive prayer requests every week through the Internet site at www.cancerprayerday.com from around the world. It is a privilege to reach out to so many people who are challenged with cancer and to touch their lives through prayer.

While we cannot address here all the philosophical and theological issues involved in the origin of disease and death, I want to point out the choices we have to become responsible to natural laws as well as spiritual principles that will help us to govern our potential health.

Making Right Choices

Lifestyle

First, we have discussed our responsibility for making lifestyle choices that will nurture our bodies, minds and spirits in health. There are natural laws that govern the health of our entire being that, when violated, guarantee that sickness will result. For example, the simple requirements that our bodies have for sleep, fresh air and water must be provided, or we will experience the consequences of sickness.

The foods we eat and the exercise we get on a regular basis will also determine our well-being. Over time, these choices we make to be responsible or irresponsible in abiding by the natural laws governing our health will determine whether we become victims of sickness. Cancer, cardiovascular diseases, obesity, diabetes and high blood pressure—the five major killers in developed countries—are all directly related to poor diet and lack of exercise. By abiding by sound dietary principles, we can reduce the risk of major illness.

Awareness

Choosing to become aware of factors outside of our immediate control that govern our health will help us to preclude their full impact on our lives. These factors include heredity, the polluted environment and accidents that can damage our immune systems or other vital organs. Stress and other mental and emotional problems that have been proven to affect our physical health must be addressed in a responsible way as well.

Obedience

Of course, there is the biblical reality that some diseases are brought upon man directly by God as a judgment for disobedience to His laws. Though this is not a popular belief for twenty-first-century Christians, it is biblical. Nothing is more displeasing to God than disobedience. The chosen people of Israel again and again tested God's tolerance with their disobedience. Here is how He responded:

> If you do not carefully follow all the words of this law, which are written in this book, and do not revere this glorious and awesome name—the LORD your God—the LORD will send fearful plagues on you and your descendants, harsh and prolonged disasters, and severe and lingering illnesses. He will bring upon you all the diseases of Egypt that you dreaded, and they will cling to you.
>
> —DEUTERONOMY 28:58–60, NIV

I personally believe that the potential for disease and death was originally released into the world through sin indiscriminately. In other words, sin brought disequilibrium to all of humanity. Sin is like a chemical plant that disposes of its toxic waste into the river—the whole community is affected. In that same way, disease will eventually affect all of us.

Yet, in my opinion, the vast majority of health problems are directly related to the *choices* we make in our everyday lives through conscious or unconscious carelessness. Even inheritance is not to blame. So we conclude that there is a cause for sickness outside of the natural order. Who then is to blame? Perhaps, to a significant extent, we are, as a result of our poor choices.

The Bible also challenges to make the right choices regarding life:

> I call heaven and earth to witness against you today, that I have set before you life and death, the blessing and the curse. So choose life in order that you may live, you and your descendants.
>
> —DEUTERONOMY 30:19

Having addressed the issue of our responsibility to protect and maintain health through proper choices as well as living in obedience to the laws of God, we still have not answered the most painful question of all: *Why me?* If millions of people are making poor choices regarding health every day, and most seem untouched by serious illness, why am I suffering a terminal diagnosis? I will try to give you the hope and help I have given many of my own patients.

Why Me?

Hindsight, without question, is always 20/20. But how do we deal with the present pain of a disease like cancer and the uncertainty of the immediate future? My heart aches for the dear people who ask the question, "Why me? Why not the serial killer who has been on death row for a couple of decades?"

Recently I was on a radio program being interviewed about prayer in medicine. I received many calls praising the fact that, as a doctor, I was promoting prayer in medical practice. But one hurting caller blurted out, "Yeah, but try praying to a God who gave you a child, an only child, with cerebral palsy." Then he hung up.

A number of my patients have asked me to explain why illness struck them. They tell me how they have led a relatively stress-free life, have tried to keep God's commandments, eaten right and exercised. When faced with death, these patients ask why this is happening if the Bible promises healing.

Helping my patients transition from fear and doubt to true spiritual freedom and trust is one of my treatment goals. They cannot be free and victorious even if they are healed of cancer but continue to fear it. Fear is as real an enemy as cancer. I help them redefine victory over cancer. Victory over the disease is not determined by whether or not they live or die; it is determined by how they live out the days that God gives them to live on the earth.

Patch Adams told me once that "the worst cancer is being alive and not enjoying life—not feeling gratitude, not loving, not living." We should not fear a medical diagnosis; we should fear not living—really living—the rest of our life, regardless of the time it may span. If God blesses you with the miracle of a cure, even if the oncologist didn't see Him roaming the hospital halls, enjoy it, be grateful, love it and live it up; nevertheless, we must all prepare for what comes next—death that ushers us into eternal life, hopefully with God.

Accepting this larger picture of life and defining true victory help us to answer the hard questions. In a very real sense, physical healing and health is, at best, temporary. From the moment we are born, technically, we begin to die. Every human being who has ever lived is in the process of dying or has already died. True and permanent healing is the condition of being in perfect balance with the Creator and His creation. That wonderful state of being cannot happen here on earth; it will occur in that infinite place some of us call heaven. Only then will health be eternal.

Grasping the significance of eternal life has more to do with temporal healing than you might realize. Many of my elderly patients recover while some of my younger patients do not. I believe the key difference between them is that the elderly patients more readily adopt the carefree attitude that says, "Whatever God wants to do is fine with me." This restful attitude frees them from stress, which plays a major factor in serious illness. The younger patients are more frequently filled with desperation to live. The stress caused by this attitude in their fight for life turns out to be counterproductive.

Another negative factor to the "Why me?" response is that when a person demands an answer to this painful question, it often drives a wedge between that individual and a caring God. The person takes his or her eyes off God and focuses only on their plight. If no answer is forthcoming, they become filled with doubt of the love of God. Left unchecked, that doubt can result in anger and even hatred toward God.

When this happens, the person's physical malignancy crosses over into the spiritual realm and becomes a malignancy of the soul. Whether or not you believe in heaven or that disease is of the devil, the outcome of a malignant attitude of doubt, anger and hatred toward your Creator will be destructive to your soul and your body. I believe this is the ultimate victory for cancer, when the physical malignancy spreads to the soul. Then, even while still living, death abides in the patient.

That does not mean we cannot resist illness or that we have to acquiesce to its ultimate fate without question. I don't believe that God wants us to passively accept an evil fate. Hezekiah, an Old Testament king, received a word from a prophet of God that he was going to die. Hezekiah rolled over in bed and cried out to God to change His plans and let him live. God heard his prayer and extended his life. (See 2 Kings 20.)

In the New Testament a blind man who heard Jesus passing by cried out so loudly that the people told him to be quiet. They were sure the Master had no time for him. Instead, he cried louder until Jesus heard and commanded them to bring the man to Him. In His mercy, He healed the man of his blindness.

I believe that our passion to reach out for help from the Master is a necessary key to our healing. Christ certainly didn't chide the blind man for not accepting his "fate." He took time to heal him miraculously. I do not believe we have to give in to illness without negotiating our situation with a caring God.

But I would admonish all to be careful with your demands to the Lord of lords. He is absolutely sovereign. Only when we are willing to see the greater picture, the eternal perspective, can we understand the enormity of God's grace in sending His only Son to die for our sins that we may live eternally in heaven. Knowing that God is in control for our good, always doing what is best

Total liberation from cancer is acknowledging that sickness, no matter how painful or grotesque, is only a moment in the eternal scheme of God.

for us, will make us victorious against disease and every other challenge of life.

For some people, victory over cancer lies in long-term prevention. For others, victory depends on finding the cure—without it their situation appears hopeless. For still others, there may be an inexplicable healing that is the result of nothing less than divine intervention of a caring God.

If you are cancer free because the disease has not stricken you, be thankful. Also, live responsibly. Do what you can to prevent it, and above all, acknowledge that by the grace of God you are enjoying the gift of health. If you are cancer free through successful treatment, be thankful to your doctor and to the source of the doctor's healing power—God. If your cancer has miraculously vanished, don't thank the heavens, circumstances or fate; thank God for His generous gift of life.

If you have recently been diagnosed with cancer, I pray that God will fill you with His grace and provide the miracle for which you are waiting and praying. Even if you do not believe in God, expect a miracle. For whether you believe in Him or not, God is a God of mercy. He desires to show you mercy.

For those of you who are veteran cancer warriors, who feel tired of the uphill battle, who have had too many disappointments and who are certain that the hope is an illusion, let me challenge your desperation and pessimism. The famous English author Samuel Johnson declared, "I will be conquered; I will not capitulate." Despite the tribulation you are facing, you can still choose whether you will be a victim or a victor.

If you ask me who my heroes are, I will tell you that they are my patients who found meaning in the midst of suffering. They discovered true victory. Being at peace with yourself is a wonderful experience, but when you are at peace with the One who made you, then you truly enter into "the zone"—that illusive place where everything seems perfect. There the points of reference are in places our minds cannot reach; they are places where our spirits are at home and can absorb the fullness of eternity.

Total liberation from cancer is acknowledging that sickness, no matter how painful or grotesque, is only a moment in the eternal scheme of God. The apostle Paul understood these eternal realities when he wrote:

> If we live, we live for the Lord, or if we die, we die for the Lord; therefore whether we live or die, we are the Lord's.
>
> —ROMANS 14:8

Again, Paul declared:

> Who shall separate us from the love of Christ? Shall tribulation, or distress, or persecution, or famine, or nakedness, or peril, or sword? Just as it is written, "For Thy sake we are being put to death all day long; we were considered as sheep to be slaughtered."
>
> But in all these things we overwhelmingly conquer through Him who loved us. For I am convinced that neither death, nor life, nor angels, nor principalities, nor things present, nor things to come, nor powers, nor height, nor depth, nor any other created thing, shall be able to separate us from the love of God, which is in Christ Jesus our Lord.
>
> —ROMANS 8:35–39

Today, I am still entangled with the mystery of Fernando's demise. But I am comforted by the fact that he received Christ as his Savior while receiving treatment for cancer. God's message to us is one of love that makes living with Him for eternity our ultimate goal. It is my prayer that, like Fernando, you too will accept that love and enjoy eternity with God where all of our questions will finally be resolved. Life with God forever—that will be the total cure for all our ills.

Appendix A

Cancer Drugs

The following list of cancer drugs are presently being used with positive results in the treatment of specific cancer conditions:

- *Tarceva* is an antigrowth agent for cancer of the head and neck.

- *Bexxar* delivers a dose of radiation directly to the lymph system.

- *Iressa* is an antigrowth agent for lung cancer.

- *GVAX* is an immune-system booster for lung cancer.

- *Neovastat* is an antiangiogenesis agent for lung cancer.

- *Virulizin* is an immune-system booster for pancreatic cancer.

- *Celecoxib* may act to prevent colon cancer.

- *Semaxanib* is an antiangiogenesis drug for colon cancer.

Appendix B

The AIDS Dilemma

Sadly, the U.S. Agency for International Development (USAID) estimates that by the year 2110 the number of orphans due to AIDS will rise to forty million—a staggering statistic when you consider that the total population of American public school children is forty-seven million.[1]

Desperate for a solution to its national crisis, the government of South Africa announced that they were refusing to uphold legal patents for AIDS drugs due to the dire need of the people. You may realize that AIDS is at dangerous, epidemic proportions throughout Africa. South of the Sahara Desert, which stretches across northern Africa, roughly 25.3 million Africans are infected with AIDS. Every day six thousand Africans die of AIDS; another eleven thousand are infected.[2] Of South Africa's forty-five million people, 4.2 million are infected with the virus, more than in any other country.[3] And since ninety-nine cents of every one dollar spent on drugs is used to pay back expensive research, the drug industry was infuriated by South Africa's decision.

Hearings for this decision by the South African government took place on March 6, 2001 in Pretoria High Court in a lawsuit brought by thirty-nine foreign drug manufacturers against them. The drug manufacturers intended to block a law passed in 1997 that would allow the South African government to override their patents and buy life-prolonging treatments for AIDS victims at a discount from developing countries or allow production of the drugs by domestic companies.[4]

South Africa won its international legal battle on the issue, over-turning longstanding protocol for the pharmaceutical industry. As you can imagine, this left the drug industry fuming because of potential revenues lost.[5]

Evaluating the Results

What was the effect of the drug AZT on the patients? The first study of patients using the drug concluded that although AZT did not prolong the life of AIDS victims, it did improve their quality of life. This is an interesting conclusion, given the fact that the drug had been discontinued in the 1970s precisely because of its toxicity that caused severe side effects.

A clinical study conducted by Harvard University on patients in advanced stages of AIDS who used AZT noted that the "improvement of the quality of life" issue simply referred to the fact that the drug retarded the onset of typical symptoms. Nevertheless, the patient did suffer from the severe side effects of AZT therapy, which included nausea, vomiting and fatigue. It was not the answer needed to cure the AIDS virus.

Abandoning the Search

Despite the competition in the pharmaceutical industry, after barely ten years of arduous research, Merck announced that it would pull out of the race to find a drug to fight the AIDS virus, owing to the enormous mutation capacity of the virus, its resistance to antivirals and a very doubtful market. Nearly all the pharmaceutical industry, its investors and scientists abandoned its search for a cure for AIDS because of the uncertain financial benefits, forgetting about the global consequences that this epidemic could cause.

AIDS is left largely untreated in Africa because of the pharmaceutical price tag of the drugs currently available. The typical American AIDS drug treatment costs an individual between $10,000 and $15,000, far beyond the financial resources of most suffering Africans.[6]

Appendix C

Business Interests

When breakthrough discoveries are "leaked" to the media, sometimes the primary purpose for the release of the information is to increase market shares. It is a fact that much research being done today is not for the betterment of mankind, but in the interest of big business. Your health issues have become big business.

Great institutions of learning have gotten into the business of research science. Today, a powerful struggle exists between institutional and private scientists. Once bastions of pure scientific pursuit, institutions such as Harvard Medical School and many others have been getting into the big business of medical research, vying for the windfall dollars it can bring.

The big business of science was once the sole proprietorship of private, for-profit pharmaceutical companies. Over the past two decades, research colleges and universities around the world have begun crossing the line from educational pursuits to big business interests. The Pasteur Institute in France was one of the largest research centers in the world. Today, Harvard School of Medicine has become the second largest profit-making center of scientific research in the world, and may soon be the largest.[1]

Most universities no longer hide the fact that they are business partners in the development of products and claim a share in patents and earnings. Sumner Slichter of Harvard University expressed it eloquently: "The discovery that an enormous amount of research can be carried on for profit is surely one of the most revolutionary economic discoveries of the century."[2]

Statements like these raise troubling questions: Does such financial pressure influence the results and data of testing? How does this possibility affect the product? The consumer? The patient? These questions beg answers to restore credibility to the medical community.

Promoting Pills—the Big Business of Marketing Pharmacology

The pharmaceutical industry leaves nothing to chance. It relies on a team of experts to constantly visit doctors and enlighten them with incontrovertible scientific studies that prove the effectiveness of their products. In the United States, the pharmaceutical industry invests billions of dollars a year promoting its pharmaceuticals.

How much will these investments yield in revenue? Let's consider the drug *Valium*, the number one prescription drug in the United States, which is prescribed for an estimated sixty million people annually. Prescription narcotics, Valium and others, kill more people than those distributed by illegal drug dealers. In the United States, thirty thousand people die annually from adverse reactions to narcotics—licit and illicit. In 1995, 7,800 (26 percent) of the deaths were victims of illegal drugs. The other 22,200 (74 percent) were patients who died from drugs that were legally prescribed.[3]

Cleaning House

Pressured by the public, the FDA began in 1972 to evaluate over-the-counter drugs, especially those of doubtful effectiveness. The immense job of reviewing 2,486 therapeutic preparations with 875 active ingredients has been very tedious, according to a reporter for *U.S. News and World Report*. More than twenty years later, only 70 percent had been evaluated.[4]

Many are a real threat to the public, and yet few have been "withdrawn."

Lamentably, the FDA still has not reviewed 30 percent of the over-the-counter drugs. It will take them many more years to get to these less toxic drugs for evaluation of their continued safety. Will the FDA ever get around to reevaluating the real toxic drugs, those that require a prescription? In the rare cases when the FDA has withdrawn a product from the market, it has usually been in response to media pressure or lawsuits.

Getting Around a Drug Ban

The pharmaceutical industry has a number of ways to get around a legislated ban of a dangerous product. One way is called off-loading or *dumping*. This is when a company targets a new international health market for a particular drug that has been banned at home. Often the new market is a Third World country where laws are weak or where officials can even be bribed.

For example, *Buscapine* was prohibited in the United States because it was considered extremely noxious. However, in Mexico, dispensing it has never been prohibited.

Incredibly, when the authorities of the FDA prohibit the sale of some product for its toxicity, it only prohibits its *distribution* in the United States; it does not prohibit its production. For example, chemical companies export DDT and other pesticides that are banned in the U.S., selling them to Mexico and other South American countries. The data concerning the dangers of many of these off-loaded products is overwhelming. In addition, Americans get the ill effects of DDT back into their stores in the low-cost produce imported from underdeveloped countries.

Appendix D

Consequences of the System

Much of the catastrophic results of drug use recorded are not available to the general public. The following cases will serve as a few painful examples:

A classic example is that of *DES*, diethylstilbestrol, which is a synthetic female hormone prescribed to halt miscarriages. DES was used extensively from the 1940s to the 1970s, despite it having been shown to cause cancer in rats. Thirty years later, the daughters of those who took DES exhibited an extraordinarily high incidence of vaginal, cervical and breast cancer, as well as liver damage. Some of their children suffered congenital deformities. These grave secondary effects persisted for two generations.[1]

In 1971, Dr. Arthur L. Herbst of Harvard University reported that not only was it not useful as an anti-abortive, but also that it was carcinogenic and caused abnormalities in unborn children. Nevertheless, it continued to be prescribed as a "day after" contraceptive and to stop the flow of breast milk, according to Robert Mendelsohn. It may surprise you to know that DES is still prescribed today.[2]

Flagyl is an antibiotic popularly prescribed by internists and surgeons. Nevertheless, it's been shown to be carcinogenic, or cancer causing. Yet, there is no indication that authorities plan to withdraw it from the market.[3]

From May 1979 to January 1980, the Smith-Kline Company released a drug on the market to treat hypertension called *Selacryn* after compliance with the FDA's rigorous norms. It caused thirty-six deaths and liver and kidney damage in many other users. The laboratory denied that there was any relationship between these incidences and the product. But courts determined that the scientists who created the drug were responsible for not reporting the evidence of risk of liver and kidney damage to the FDA, and the laboratory lost its case.[4]

Among the drugs prescribed most often are those used to combat high blood pressure. Hypertension generally develops in poorly nourished men and women who are under stress. Talk about market opportunity in our high-pressure society! Merck produces one of the most popular hypertension medications, with annual sales topping at about one $100 million.[5]

And although it is true that antihypertension drugs can help bring down your blood pressure, they do not reduce mortality from heart attacks or blood clots. That means that the individuals who take these medications have the same mortality rate as those who do not. Besides being an unnecessary expense, their side effects include headaches, nausea and impotence.

The Children's Market

Not even the children are spared from the drug market blitz. Every day more and more cases of hyperactivity and ADD are diagnosed among children. *Dexedrine, Cylert, Ritalin* and *Tofranil* are prescribed for these youngsters. Yet, few of these parents realize that these medications can damage the brain, sometimes permanently, or that they could solve many of their children's problems with some simple dietary changes.[6]

Junk food is a major cause of behavioral problems in children. The negative effects of these ADD and hyperactivity medications are high blood pressure, nervousness and sleeplessness, as well as disturbed growth. Children taking these drugs show less disposition to respond to stimuli, lose their sense of humor and become apathetic. Nor have these drugs been shown to help children learn better at school; on the contrary, the children act like zombies.[7]

In the case of Ritalin, the children may become withdrawn, no longer making "trouble for their teachers or get into fights, they begin to exist in a state of disconnected social isolation." Or they show the opposite effect; they become more agitated.[8]

Appendix E

Modern Research Proves
Significance of Diet

Gerald Keusch and other researchers found that "nutritional status plays a critical role in immunological defense mechanisms at a number of important levels."[1]

Researcher Robert Good and others agreed that nutritional factors "can have profound influences on...the development and manifestations of cancers" as well as other diseases.[2]

In his research, Eduardo Siguel outlines a diet much the same as Gerson's as being the ideal way to strengthen the body's immune system against cancerous cells. His ideal diet was high in carbohydrates and vegetables and low in protein.[3]

Appendix F

Contamination of Water Supplies

In the year 1956, a dramatic case of food poisoning occurred in the region of the Bay of Minamata, Japan. The problem was traced to a factory that dumped untreated waste into the ocean. One hundred twenty-one persons were poisoned when they ate contaminated crustaceans and mollusks. Forty percent of these victims died from cerebral lesions.

A more shocking example took place in 1940 with the birth of the petrochemical industry. Scientists discovered how to produce synthetic products, a discovery that promised to lower costs and introduce thousands of useful products for consumers. In that year, one billion pounds of chemically synthetic substances that had never been seen in nature were produced. In the following decade, production rose to fifty billion pounds, and by the 1980s half a trillion pounds.[1] Obviously it was impossible for governmental agencies to investigate each one of the chemical substances created to determine their level of toxicity.

In the United States, there are four million recognized chemical compounds. This number increases each year by approximately one thousand new products.[2] The time and cost of laboratory tests makes it impossible to keep up with production. Millions of substances have not been tested, yet it is known that some six hundred of them are highly carcinogenic. It took three decades and $40 million to unequivocally prove that tobacco causes cancer.[3] The producers of cigarettes relied on huge economic resources to counteract these investigations. Just imagine the vast resources of the petrochemical industry! Meanwhile these chemicals and their by-products are spoiling the soil and the water.

In 1972, the United States initiated a program to build sewage treatment plants throughout the nation. Unfortunately, water treatment plants cannot even detect, much less detoxify, most of the chemical substances that are dumped into the water. Present methods of treatment consist of filtering out dangerous waste from known sources of contaminants. This is a good start, but in reality new contaminants escape even the most modern filtration systems. A survey of tap water reserves in the United States in 954 cities revealed that 30 percent are contaminated, while seventeen pesticides have been found in the groundwater of twenty-three states.[4]

It is calculated that the chemical industry in the United States produces sixty thousand highly toxic compounds that end up in the water supply.[5] The government claims to enforce laws that prohibit the production of many of these substances. However, it is well known that chemical plants are not effectively monitored.

Appendix G

Nuclear Contamination

Hard lessons about nuclear toxins were learned by the residents of Love Canal, an industrial county in New York where one of the largest dumps of nuclear waste exists. Researchers reported the following health hazards for those who live near the site:

- The rate of involuntary abortion is three times the national average.

- Fifty-six percent of the county's children suffer from both physical and mental deficiencies.

- The incidence of cancer is three times greater than the rest of the country.[1]

The Nuclear Arms Race

During the Cold War, the world was held hostage by fears of global annihilation by nuclear weapons. Although war between superpowers no longer preoccupies our thoughts, the fallout of that era has never ceased. More than one thousand atomic bombs are said to have been detonated on American soil in military tests.[2] The toxic effects of this testing is staggering.

After an explosion, atoms of uranium and plutonium produce hundreds of radioactive particles called isotopes. This radioactive material is trapped in the atmosphere, where it eventually falls back down to earth as radioactive rain. All living creatures are very sensitive to radioisotopes. They invade our bodies through the air, water and contaminated foods. Even though some of them are fleeting, most will stay in the earth forever. For instance, the average life of carbon-14, a radioactive particle, is 5,760 years!

On April 26, 1986 in Chernobyl, Ukraine, the world was shaken by the worst nuclear industrial accident in history. The explosion contaminated the atmosphere with 100 million curies of radioisotopes that expanded from the Ukraine to Great Britain.[3] Only thirty-one persons died in the explosion, but it would be impossible to calculate the resultant deaths from the radiation released from the accident.

Ten thousand deer in Europe ate feed that had been contaminated from radioactive rain following the disaster and died as a result.[4] Europeans were also bathed in this rain, as well as their crops and soil. The long-term effects of exposure to small doses of radiation can last for many decades.[5]

One of these nuclear contaminants, strontium-90, is an isotope that easily contaminates milk. Where humans and animals are exposed to it, leukemia and bone cancer levels increase dramatically.[6]

Mormons have enjoyed a low incidence of cancer because they avoid the consumption of caffeine, alcohol and tobacco. Ironically, the incidence of cancer has increased among them in spite of their dietary consideration. That is likely because many of them live in Utah, close to atomic test sites. Victims of Hiroshima and Nagasaki have an extraordinarily high rate of cancer. But malignancies are not the only health hazard; they also suffer from small skulls and functionally impaired brains.

One of the most threatening risks of radiation is that of mutations. Almost all radioactive materials can induce genetic mutations. Before protection against radiation was so sophisticated, tests were made on the families of two thousand radiologists. These studies revealed that the index of fetal deaths and congenital deformities was higher for those exposed to radiation than the rest of the population.

Activists want nuclear energy plants to be dismantled for the threat they are to our world, but most of the radiation we receive comes naturally from the sun and other natural sources in the water, soil and atmosphere. Ten percent of the radiation to which we are exposed comes from nuclear plants, and 90 percent comes from the medical industry through x-rays, nuclear medicine and radiation therapy.

Appendix H

Issels' Cancer Treatment: A Technical Discussion

Dr. Issels' essential programs included research on pleomorphism (Enderlein) and microbes in oncogenesis, for example, mycoplasma (Gerlach), autologous vaccines (Coley), darkfield microscopy, hyperthermia, etc.

Dr. Issels differentiated between two causal complexes in the development of cancer, namely:

- The factors that induce the transformation of a normal cell into a cancer cell

- Those factors that impair the immune and regulatory systems to an extent that they cannot prevent cancer cells from developing into a tumor.

Based on the holistic concept, the Issels Treatment has two main lines of approach to cancer that complement each other.

I. Treatment aiming at the removal or reduction of the tumor
   A. Surgery
   B. Radiation
   C. Chemotherapy
   D. Hormone Therapy
   E. Hyperthermia and other nontoxic modalities
   F. Specific immunotherapy

II. Nonspecific immunobiological basic treatment aimed at the restoration of the impaired defense, repair and regulatory functions of the tumor host

211

A. Elimination of all sizable exogenous and endogenous casual factors that may lead to an impairment of the immune functions and may contribute to a transformation of the symbiotic microorganisms into pathogens
   1. Malnutrition to be replaced by a diet designed to meet the special needs of the individual cancer patient (Budwig, Gerson, Hildenbrand), with supplementation of vitamins, antioxidants, minerals, trace elements, enzymes
   2. Abnormal bacterial intestinal flora to be normalized by diet and long-term administration of *coli* cultures (Nissle) and other probiotic cultures
   3. Head foci of infection such as dental, alveolar and tonsillar foci to be removed by surgical intervention (Issels, Pischinger)
   4. Fields of neural disturbance to be neutralized by neural therapy (Huneke). Neural therapy and acupuncture are also administered in conjunction with conventional therapy.
   5. Hereditary allergoses and toxicoses to be treated by administration of specific colloids (Issels, Spengler)
   6. Environmental and occupational factors and addictions to be rectified by change in lifestyle
   7. Psychic stress to be relieved by psychological guidance, in single and group therapy, biofeedback, relaxation techniques, meditation and visualization
   8. Physical therapy, hydrotherapy, breathing techniques, massage, lymph drainage and so forth
B. Treatment of secondary damage and metabolic disturbance to restore normal function of organs by:
   1. Activation of cellular respiration by oxygen-ozone therapy in various forms, ultraviolet blood irradiation
   2. Regeneration of organs and compensation of losses by administration of organ extracts or organ hydrolysates (e.g., liver extract, thymus peptides)
   3. Therapy to improve detoxification, i.e., elimination of toxins resulting from oncolysis and of metabolic residues by activation of liver and kidney function

assisted by herbal extracts and high fluid intake, colon-hydrotherapy, enemas

4. Enzyme therapy with lytic enzymes to eliminate immune suppressive factors such as immune complexes
5. Homeopathy, Isopathy

C. Stimulation of immune response by hyperpyrexia, i.e., the injection of bacterial lypopolysaccharides, e.g., an autolysate of streptococci and bacterium prodigiosum (Coley), to raise body temperature up to 105° F. Hyperpyrexia fights latent infections, loosens regulative blockades, improves detoxification, damages cancer cells, temporarily raises the white blood count up to 30–40,000 and increases the release of interferon and interleukin. (Over the past forty years more than one hundred applications were given in the Issels Hospital and Clinic in Germany without any adverse side effects.)

1. Biological response modifiers, autologous vaccines

The vaccines were developed in the Microbiological Department of the Issels Hospital. From 1958 until 1973 Dr. Franz Gerlach was its director of research. He was professor of the University of Vienna, a researcher of the Pasteur Institute in Paris, well published in peer-reviewed medical journals and internationally renowned for his research on mycoplasma and cancer.

Especially during the first years of the development of the Issels Treatment, it became evident: Specific immunotherapy was more effective when casual factors could be eliminated systematically and detoxification mechanisms and herewith the endogenous environment, the "melliu" could be normalized.

The normalization of the detoxification process is an essential part of basic therapy. This is generally ignored in research and practice. Despite all efforts, even today, many patients are lost who respond well to the tumor antigens, but who are not able to excrete the products of tumor lysis.

Without sufficient detoxification neither immunotherapy nor chemotherapy will achieve long-term results.

In patients with a rapidly growing tumor who cannot expect immediate help from long-term immunotherapy, the latter is combined with chemotherapy according to the morphology of the tumor. Thus the progression of the tumor growth can be stopped and the patient gains time to respond to immunotherapy.

It has also observed that through comprehensive immunobiological treatment alone or in combination with chemotherapy, a variety of inoperable tumors can be rendered operable. Blocked ureters or gall-bladders can be freed, making it possible to continue treatment of patients who would otherwise be lost.

Dr. Issels believed that cancer is a systemic disease, one that affects the entire body but manifests in a particular location where a tumor develops. Tumors are caused by factors inside and outside of an individual's body that create mutations, sensitize or cause neural effects that then damage organs and organ systems and cause functional disturbances of the neural, hormonal, excretory and defense systems.[1]

Notes

Introduction: We Will Win Against Cancer!

1. American Cancer Society, *Cancer Facts and Figures* (Atlanta: American Cancer Society, 2002), 2.
2. Ernesto Contreras Sr., *To You, My Beloved Patient* (Chula Vista, CA: Interpacific Press, 1999), 64–65.
3. Francisco Contreras, *Health in the 21ˢᵗ Century: Will Doctors Survive?* (Chula Vista, CA: Interpacific Press, 1997), 130.

Chapter 1: A Paradigm for Cancer Treatment

1. J. Hill, *Cautions Against the Immoderate Use of Snuff* (London: Baldwin & Jackson, 1761), 27–38.
2. S. T. Soemmerring, *De Morbis Vasorum Absorbentium Corporis Humani* (Frankfurt, Germany: Varrentrapp and Wenner, 1795), 109.
3. E. F. Bouisson, *Tribut a la Chirurgie* (Paris: Balliere, 1858), 1259–1303.
4. Robert N. Proctor, "Tobacco and the Global Lung Cancer Epidemic," *Nature Reviews: Cancer*, vol. 1 (October 2001).
5. M. Kaminsky, Thesis: *Ein Primares Lungencarcinom mit Verhornte Plattenepithelien* (University of Greifswald, 1898).
6. R. Kluger, *Ashes to Ashes: America's Hundred-Year Cigarette War, the Public Health, and the Unabashed Triumph of Phillip Morris* (New York: Knopf, 1996), 13.
7. Proctor, "Tobacco and the Global Lung Cancer Epidemic," 86.
8. Ibid., 82.
9. World Health Organization, *Tobacco and Health: A Global Status Report* (Geneva: World Health Organization, 1999).
10. American Cancer Society, *Cancer Facts and Figures*, 4. Source obtained from the Internet: Surveillance Research, www.cancer.org
11. George Crile Jr., *The Way It Was—Sex, Surgery, Treasure and Travel 1907-1987* (Kent, Ohio: Kent State University Press, 1992).
12. Bernard Fisher and C. Redmond, *Studies of the National Surgical Adjuvant Project* (Amsterdam: Elservier/North Holland: Biomedical Press, 1977), 67–81.
13. Ibid.
14. Crile Jr., *The Way It Was—Sex, Surgery, Treasure and Travel*

        1907–1987.
15.   Source obtained from the Internet: www.uhealthnet.on.ca/library archives.htm.
16.   Fisher and Redmond, *Studies of the National Surgical Adjuvant Project.*
17.   Crile Jr., *The Way It Was—Sex, Surgery, Treasure and Travel 1907–1987.*
18.   "The chemo's Berlin wall crumbles," *Cancer Chronicles* (December 1990): 4
19.   Ibid.
20.   Ibid.
21.   Marion Morra and Eve Potts, *Realistic Alternatives in Cancer Treatment* (New York: Avon Books, 1980), 176.
22.   Ibid.

Chapter 2: A Paradigm Shift in Cancer Treatment

1.   *Cancer,* 1990.
2.   Ibid.
3.   T. Boveri, *"mehrpoige mitosen ais mittel zur analyse des zellkerns,"* Verh. D. Phys. Med. Ges., Wurzberg N.F. 35 (1902): 67–90.
4.   T. Boveri, *Zur Frage der Enstenhung Maligner Tumoren* (Gustav Fisher: Jena, 1914), 1–64.
5.   Michael D. Lemonick and Alice Park, "New Hope for Cancer," *Time* (May 28, 2001): 66–67.
6.   Ibid.
7.   M. L. Pardue and P. G. DeBaryshe, "Telomeres and telomerase: more than the end of the line," *Chromosoma* 108 (1999): 73–82.
8.   Source obtained from the Internet: "Cellular Fountain of Youth Works, Scientists Conclude," (January 13, 1998): www.mercurycenter.com/scitech.center/agingo1498.
9.   T. M. Nakamura et al., "Telomerase catalytic subunit homologs from fission yeast and human," *Science* 277 (1997): 955–959. M. Meyerson et al., "HEST2 the putative human telomerase catalytic subunit gene, is up-regulated n tumor cells and during immortalization," *Cell* 90 (1997): 785–795. A. G. Bodnar et al., "Extension of life-span by introduction of telomerase into normal human cells," *Science* 279 (1998): 349–352. H. Vaziri and S. Benchimol, "Reconstitutions of telomerase activity in normal human cells leads to elongation of telomeres and extended replicative life span," *Curr. Biol.* 8 (1998): 279–282.
10.   Allan Balmain, "Cancer genetics: from Boveri and Mendel to microarrays," *Nature Reviews: Cancer,* vol. 1 (October 2001): 77.
11.   D. Stehelin, H. E. Varmus, J. M. Bishop and P. K. Vogt, "DNA related

to the transforming gene(s) of avian sarcoma viruses is present in normal avian DNA," *Nature* 260 (1976): 170–173. J. M. Bishop, "Enemies within: the genesis of retrovivral oncogenes," *Cell* 23 (1981): 5–6.

12. Balmain, "Cancer genetics: from Boveri and Mendel to microarrays," 78.
13. bid.
14. Ibid., 77. C. Shih et al., "Passage of phenotypes of chemically transformed cells via transfection of DNA and chromatin," *Proc. Natl. Acad. Sci. USA* 11 (1979): 5714–5718.
15. A. Balmain and I. B. Pragnell, "Mouse skin carcinomas induced in vivo by chemical carcinogens have a transforming Harvey-ras oncogene," *Nature* 303: 72–74.
16. S. Sukumar, V. Notario, D. Martin-Zanca, A. Balmain et al., "Carcinogen-specific mutation and amplification of the Ha-ras gene during mouse skin carcinogenesis," *Nature* 322 (1986): 78–80.
17. Balmain, "Cancer genetics: from Boveri and Mendel to microarrays," 78.
18. Ibid.
19. Boveri, *"mehrpoige mitosen ais mittel zur analyse des zellkerns,"* 1–64.
20. Ibid.
21. A. G. Knudson Jr., "Mutations and cancer: statistical study of retinoblastoma," *Proc. Natl Acad. Sci. USA* 68 (1971): 820–823.
22. Balmain, "Cancer genetics: from Boveri and Mendel to microarrays," 79.
23. W. K. Cavenee et al., "Expression of recessive alleles by chromosomal mechanisms in retinoblastoma," *Nature* 305 (1983): 779–781.
24. J. Groden et al., "Identification and characterization of the familial adenomatous polyposis coli gene," *Cell* 66 (1991): 589–600. I. Nishisho et al., "Mutations of chromosomes 5q21 genes in FAP and colorectal cancer patients," *Science* 253 (1991): 665–669. K.W. Kinzler et al., "Identification of FAP locus genes from chromosomes 5q21," *Science* 253 (1991): 661–665. P. A. Futreal et al., "BRCA1 mutations in primary breast and ovarian carcinomas," *Science* 266 (1994): 120–122. Y. Miki et al., "A strong candidate for the breast and ovarian cancer susceptibility gene BRCA1," *Science* 266 (1994): 66–71.
25. Cavenee et al., "Expression of recessive alleles by chromosomal mechanisms in retinoblastoma." S. H. Friend et al., "A human DNA segment with properties of the gene that predisposes to retinoblastoma and osteosarcoma," *Nature* 334 (1986): 643–646.

Chapter 3: A Brave New World of Cancer Drugs

1. John Cary, "This Drug's for You: Genetically Tailored Treatments Could Transform Medicine," reprinted from *Business Week* (January 18, 1999) and *Continental* (March 1999): 51–53.
2. Michael C. Lemonic and Alice Park, "There Is New Ammunition in the War Against Cancer," *Time* (May 28, 2001): 64.
3. Ibid.
4. Cary, "This Drug's for You: Genetically Tailored Treatments Could Transform Medicine."
5. Lemonick and Park, "New Hope for Cancer," 65.
6. Ibid., 64.
7. Ibid.
8. Ibid., 65.
9. Ibid., 66.
10. Ibid., 65.
11. Ibid., 67.
12. Ibid., 68.
13. Ibid.

Chapter 4: Caution: Following the Money Trail

1. Lemonick and Park, "New Hope for Cancer," 69.
2. Barry Werth, *The Billion-Dollar Molecule: One Company's Quest for the Perfect Drug* (New York: Simon and Schuster, 1994), 268.
3. Ibid.
4. Ibid., 269.
5. Joseph D. Beasley, *The Betrayal of Health: The impact of nutrition, environment and lifestyle on illness in America* (New York: Random House, 1991), 199.
6. Eustace Mullins, *Murder by Injection USA* (The National Council of Medical Research, 1998), 101.
7. Ibid.
8. American Cancer Society, *Cancer Facts and Figures*, 2.
9. Source obtained from the Internet: American Cancer Society, *Cancer Facts and Figures 2001*, Surveillance Research, 2001, www.cancer.org.

Chapter 5: Exciting Cancer Treatments: Laetrile; Issels' Therapy

1. Source obtained from the Internet: www.worldwithoutcancer.com/ hunza.
2. Source obtained from the Internet: Gregory M. Fahy, "Aging

Revealed," Life Foundation, http://lef.org/magazine/mag99/nov99-cover.

3. Source obtained from the Internet: Jane Kinderlehrer; "Death Rides a Slow Bus in Hunza," www.millenicom.com/~markstickels/longhealthylife/Hunzaland.

4. Ibid.

5. Source obtained from the Internet: www.worldwithoutcancer.com/hunza.

6. Ibid.

7. G. Edward Griffin, *World Without Cancer* (Westlake Village, CA: American Media, 1997), 85–95.

8. Source obtained from the Internet: www.worldwithoutcancer.com/hunza.

9. Source obtained from the Internet: www.encyclopedia.com/articles/13588.

10. For more information about the Oasis of Hope Hospital and treatments available there, visit our website at www.oasisofhope.com.

Chapter 6: Ozone Therapy: A Potential Cure

1. Otto Warburg, *The Metabolism of Tumors*, tr. F. Dickens (London, 1930).

2. B. Bocci, "Is ozone therapy therapeutic?," *Perspectives in Biology and Medicine* 42 (1998): 131–143.

3. V. Bocci, N. Di Paolo, G. Garosi, C. Aldinucci, E. Borrelli, G. Valacchi, F. Cappelli, L. Guerri, G. Gavioli, F. Corradeschi, R. Rossi, F. Giannerini and P. Di Simplicio P, Preliminary studies, *International Journal of Artificial Organs* 22(9) (1999): 645–651.

4. "Ozone Selectively Inhibits Growth of Human Cancer Cells," *Science* 209 (22 August 1980): 931–933.

Chapter 7: Gerson's Empirical Evidence for Diet Therapy

1. Source obtained from the Internet: www.gerson.org/index.shtml.

2. Ferninand Sauerbruch, *Master Surgeon* [*Das War Mein Leben*] (London: Andre Deutsch, 1953), 167–171.

3. Max Gerson, *Diet Therapy of Lung Tuberculosis* [*Diatbehandlung der Tuberkulose*] (Leipzig and Vienna: Franz Deuticke, 1934).

4. Patricia Spain Ward, *History of the Gerson Therapy: Contract report prepared for the U.S. Office of Technology Assessment* (Washington, DC: U.S. Government Printing Office, 1988).

5. Ibid.

6. Ibid.

7. Max Gerson, M.D., "The cure of advanced cancer by diet therapy: a summary of 30 years of clinical experimentation," *Physiol Chem Phys* 10(5) (1978): 449–464.

8. Max Neuburger, "An Historical Study of the Concept of Nature from a Medical viewpoint," *Issi* 3s (1944): 16–28. John Harley Warner, "The Nature-Trusting Heresy; American Physicians and the Concept of the Healing Power of Nature in the 1850 and 1860s," *Perspectives in American History* 11 (1978): 291–324. Ward, "History of the Gerson therapy."

9. Max Gerson, M.D., *A Cancer Therapy: Results of 50 Cases* (New York: Whittier Books, 1958).

10. Ward, "History of the Gerson therapy."

11. Guy R. Newell and Neil M. Ellison, eds., *Nutrition and Cancer: Etiology and Treatment* (New York: Raven Press, 1981).

12. G. N. Ling, "The Association Induction Hypothesis: A Theoretical Foundation Provided for the Possible Beneficial Effects of a Low Sodium, High Potassium Diet and Other Similar Regimens in the Treatment of Patients Suffering from Debilitating Illnesses," *Agressologie* 24 (1983): 293–301.

13. Gerald T. Keusch, Carla S. Wilson and Samuel E. Waksal, *Nutrition, Host Defenses, and the Lymphoid System: Advances in Host Defense Mechanisms*, vol. 2, John I. Gallin and Anthony S. Fauci, eds. (New York: Raven Press, 1983).

14. Ward, "History of the Gerson therapy."

15. Ibid.

16. Ibid.

17. Ibid.

18. Paul B. Beeson, "Changes in Medical Therapy During the Past Half Century," *Medicine* 59 (1980): 79–99.

19. Charles B. Simone, *Cancer and Nutrition* (New York: McGraw-Hill Book Co., 1983) 64.

20. Ward, "History of the Gerson therapy."

21. Ibid.

22. James Rorty, *American Medicine Mobilizes* (New York: W.W. Norton & Co., Inc.; 1939).

23. Ward, "History of the Gerson therapy."

24. From Patrick Quillan, Ph.D., R.D., C.N.S., *Nature's Impact* (Oct./Nov. 1998): 47.

25. Michael Gearin-Tosch, *Living Proof: A Medical Mutiny* (New York: Simon and Schuster, n.d.), 278.

26. Source obtained from the Internet: www.hacres.com/articles.asp.

Chapter 8: The Power of Prevention—Living Foods

1. Information obtained from the Internet by searching the Guinness Book of World Records with Texis, Thunderstone Document Retrieval and Management. Also found at www.uselessfacts.net/facts/health_and_body/more8.shmtl.

2. Beasley, *The Betrayal of Health*, 85.

3. Ibid., 108.

4. Robert M. Kradjian, "Milk, the natural thing?", *Newlife* (November–December 1994).

5. Ibid.

6. Ibid.

7. Contreras, *Health in the 21ˢᵗ Century*, 107.

8. Ibid., 108.

9. Ibid.

10. Theo Colborn, *Our Stolen Future* (New York: Penguin Group, 1997), 150–152.

11. Richard M. Sharpe and Niels S. Skakkebaek, "Are estrogens involved in falling sperm counts and disorders of the male reproductive tract?", *Lancet* 341 (May 29, 1993): 1392–1395.

12. Francisco Contreras, M.D., *The Hope of Living Cancer Free* (Lake Mary, FL: Siloam Press, 1999), 98.

13. L. A. Brinton, "Ways that women may reduce their possible risk of breast cancer," *Journal of the National Cancer Institute* (1994).

14. Ralph W. Moss, Ph.D., "Cancer Risks Lurk in Hot Dogs and Burgers," *Cancer Chronicles* (July 1994).

15. Susan Preston-Martin et al., "Maternal Consumption of Cured Meats and Vitamins in Relation to Pediatric Brain Tumors," *Cancer Epidemiology, Biomarkers and Prevention* 5, 599–605.

16. Beasley, *The Betrayal of Health*, 106.

17. Julian Whitaker, M.D., *Health and Healing*, vol. 7, no. 11 (November 1977).

18. Beasley, *The Betrayal of Health*, 87.

19. Contreras, *The Hope of Living Cancer Free*, 101.

20. D. Burkett and H. Trowell, *Western Diseases and Their Emergence and Prevention* (Cambridge, MA: Harvard University Press, 1981).

21. Kian Liu et al., "Dietary cholesterol, fat, and fiber, and cancer colon mortality. An analysis of international data," *Lancet* 2 (October 13, 1979): 782–785. El Wynder, "Dietary habits and cancer epidemiology," *Cancer* 43 (5 Suppl) (May 1979): 1955–1961.

22. *Cancer Research*, 1974.

23. Stephen Shoenthaler, "Institutional Nutritional Policies and Criminal

Behavior," *Nutrition Today* 20(3) (1985): 16.

24. Stephen Shoenthaler, "Diet and Crime: An Empirical Examination of the Value of Nutrition in the Control and Treatment of Incarcerated Juvenile Offenders," *International Journal of Biosocial Research* 4(1) (1983): 25–39.

25. Beasley, *The Betrayal of Health*, 76.

26. Ibid., 77.

27. D. Lonsdale and R. J. Shamberger, "Red Cell transketolase as an indicator of nutritional deficiency," *American Journal of Clinical Nutrition* 33 (1980): 205–221. Beasley, *The Betrayal of Health*, 77.

28. A. P. Simopoulos, "The Mediterranean diets: What is so special about the diet of Greece? The scientific evidence," *J Nutr* 131, 11 Suppl. (November 2001): 3065S–3073S.

29. Nakagawa, "Resveratrol inhibits human breast cancer cell growth and may mitigate the effect of linoleic acid, a potent breast cancer cell stimulator," *J Cancer Res Clin Oncol* 127(4) (April 2001): 258–264.

30. B. D. Gehm, "Resveratrol, a polyphenolic compound found in grapes and wine, is an agonist for the estrogen receptor," *Proc Natl Acad Sci U S A* 94(25) (December 9, 1997): 14138–14143.

31. P. A. Davis, "Whole almonds and almond fractions reduce aberrant crypt foci in a rat model of colon carcinogenesis," *Cancer Lett* 165(1) (April 10, 2001): 27–33.

32. E. Giovannucci, "A prospective study of tomato products, lycopene, and prostate cancer risk," *J Natl Cancer Inst* 94(5) (March 6, 2002): 391–398.

33. M. Jang, "Cancer chemopreventive activity of resveratrol," *Drugs Exp Clin Res* 25(2–3) (1999): 65–77.

Chapter 9: Prevention Through Lifestyle

1. Source obtained from the Internet: Independence: Fitness advice by Sheila King for Underwire, resources for women, January 10, 2001; http://underwire.msn.com/Underwire/bodyworks/fm/63dispatch.asp.

2. Ibid.

3. Ibid.

4. Source obtained from the Internet: World Health Network, Longevity, Life Expectancy and Anti-aging Medicine, October 22, 1999; www.worldhealth.net/news/exercise3/html.

5. Christine Gorman, "Walk, Don't Run," *Time* (January 21, 2002).

6. Source obtained from the Internet: World Health Network, Longevity, Life Expectancy and Anti-aging Medicine, October 22, 1999; www.worldhealth.net/news/exercise3/html

7. Ibid.
8. Ibid.
9. Ibid.
10. Ibid.
11. Gorman, "Walk, Don't Run."
12. Ibid. Source obtained from the Internet: AMA Health Insight, General Health by Theodore Berland, www.ama-assn.org/Insight/Gen_Hlth/ Fittness/Fitnes2.htm: Fitness Basics, Medical Review by Jeffrey Tanji, M.D., University of California, Davis, Posted: Nov. 20, 1997.
13. Source obtained from the Internet: AFAR, News From AFAR, Weighty Issues for Seniors, www.afar.org/weight.
14. Source obtained from the Internet: World Health Network, www.worldhealth.net/news/exercise3.
15. S. Begley, "Religion and the brain," *Newsweek* 137(19) (May 7, 2001): 50–57.
16. R. A. Neimeyer, "Unfounded trust: a constructivist meditation," *Am J Psychother* 55(3) (2001): 364–371.
17. C. Shang, "Emerging paradigms in mind-body medicine," *J Altern Complement Med* 7(1) (February 2001): 83–91.
18. D. Lehmann, "Brain sources of EEG gamma frequency during volitionally meditation-induced, altered states of consciousness, and experience of the self," *Psychiatry Res* 108(2) (November 30, 2001): 111–121.
19. B. M. Jones, "Changes in cytokine production in healthy subjects practicing Guolin Qigong: a pilot study," *BMC Complement Altern Med* 1(1) (2001): 8.
20. M. Haid, "Modulation of germination and growth of plants by meditation," *Am J Chin Med* 29(3–4) (2001): 393–401.
21. F. Travis, "Physiological patterns during practice of the Transcendental Meditation technique compared with patterns while reading Sanskrit and a modern language," *Int J Neurosci* 109(1–2) (July 2001): 71–80.
22. S. R. Bishop, "What do we really know about mindfulness-based stress reduction?", *Psychosom Med* 64(1) (January–February 2002): 71–83.
23. P. G. Brolinson, "Nurses' perceptions of complementary and alternative medical therapies," *J Community Health* 26(3) (June 2001): 175–189.
24. N. E. Schoenberger, "Opinions and practices of medical rehabilitation professionals regarding prayer and meditation," *J Altern Complement Med* 8(1) (February 2002): 59–69.
25. B. J. Bernstein, "Prevalence of complementary and alternative medicine use in cancer patients," *Oncology (Hunting)* 15(10) (October 2001): 1267–1272; discussion, 1272–1278, 1283.

26. M. Haid, "Modulation of germination and growth of plants by meditation."

Chapter 10: Environment: Our Responsibility

1. Delfin García, "Veneno en la piel" (Poison in the skin), *Muy interesante* XII, no. 1, 40–46.

2. Source obtained from the Internet: Donald Sutherland, "Tug-o-War: Cancer Kids vs. Water Pollution," Environment News Service; ens.lycos.com/ens/sep99/1999L-09-27-01.html.

3. Ibid.

4. Source obtained from the Internet: www.epa.gov/safewater/hfacts.html.

5. Source obtained from the Internet: EPA Office of Environmental Information, www.epa.gov/triexplorer/chemical.htm.

6. Source obtained from the Internet: www.sima.com.mx/valle_de_mexico/introduc1.htm.

7. E. Mann, "L.A. smogbusters," *The Nation* (September 17, 1990): 254–274. Beasley, *The Betrayal of Health,* 119.

8. Source obtained from the Internet: CNN.com, Fighting deforestation of the rainforest, October 19, 2001.

9. Beasley, *The Betrayal of Health,* 120.

10. Ibid., 127.

11. Ibid., 115.

12. Source obtained from the Internet: www.epa.gov/region07/programs/spfd/nplfacts/shenandoah_stables.pdf.

13. Beasley, *The Betrayal of Health,* 127.

14. Contreras, *Health in the 21st Century,* 66–67.

15. C. J. Johnson, "Cancer incidence in an area of radioactive fallout downwind from the Nevada test site," *Journal of the American Medical Association* 251(2): 230–236. Beasley, *The Betrayal of Health,* 131.

16. Source obtained from the Internet: Tim Conner, "Nuclear workers at risk," Bulletin of the Atomic Scientists, Vol. 46, No. 8 (September 1990): www.bullatomsci.org/issues/1990/s90/s90conner.

17. American Cancer Society, *Cancer Facts and Figures* (Atlanta: American Cancer Society, 1999).

18. Beasley, *The Betrayal of Health,* 122–123.

19. A. V. Zamm, *Why Your House May Endanger Your Health* (New York: Simon and Schuster, 1982), 49. Beasley, *The Betrayal of Health,* 123.

20. Beasley, *The Betrayal of Health,* 125.

21. Ibid., 125.

22. Gabriel Quadri de la Torre, "Desarrollo sustentable. Hacia una política ambiental," Universidad Nacional Autónoma de México (1993).

Chapter 11: Weighing in With Alternative Medicine

1. David M. Eisenberg et al., "Trends in alternative medicine use in the United States, 1990–1997," *Journal of the American Medical Association* 280 (November 11, 1998): 1569–1575.

2. Source obtained from the Internet: Hans R. Larsen., MSc ChE; "Alternative Medicine: Why So Popular?", International Health News; www.yourhealthbase.com.

3. Eisenberg, "Trends in alternative medicine use in the United States, 1990–1997."

4. Alan Bensoussan, "Complementary medicine: where lies its appeal?", *Medical Journal of Australia* 170 (March 15, 1999): 247–248 (editorial). Peter Fisher and Adam Ward, "Complementary medicine in Europe," *British Medical Journal* 309 (July 9, 1994): 107–111.

5. Source obtained from the Internet: Reuters, New York; Nov. 10; 1999; submitted by Christopher Wiechert; Alternative Medicine's Popularity Is Rising; joyful@best.com.

6. Ibid.

7. Ibid.

8. Ibid.

9. Source obtained from the Internet: John Lacey; Alternative Medicine Is Here to Stay; UniSci, Daily University Science News; webmaster@unisci.com.

10. Ibid.

11. Ibid.

12. Larsen, "Alternative Medicine: Why So Popular?"

13. Ibid.

14. *The Lancet* (November 7, 1992): 1136–1139.

15. Timothy J. Wilt et al., "Saw palmetto extracts for treatment of benign prostatic hyperplasia," *Journal of the American Medical Association* 280 (November 11, 1998): 1604–1609.

16. Larsen, "Alternative Medicine: Why So Popular?"

17. Source obtained from the Internet: CSICOP/News/Scientists and Physicians Gather in Philadelphia for "Science Meets Alternative Medicine"; www.hcrc.org/sram.

18. Ibid.

19. N. Gevitz, *Other Healers: Unorthodox Medicine in America* (Baltimore, MD: The John Hopkins University Press, 1988).

20. K. D. Bagshawe, "Antibody directed enzymes revive anti-cancer pro-drug concept," *Br. J. Cancer* 56 (1987): 531–532; R. G. Melton and R. F. Sherwood, "Antibody-enzyme conjugates for cancer therapy," *J. Natl. Cancer Inst.* 88 (1996): 153–165; K. N. Syrigos and A. A.

Epenetos, "Antibody directed enzyme pro-drug therapy (ADEPT): A review of the experimental and clinical considerations," *Anticancer Res.* 19 (1999): 605–614.

21. M. S. Wetzel, D. M. Eisenburg and T. J. Kaptchuk, "Courses involving complementary and alternative medicine at U.S. medical schools," *JAMA* 280 (1998): 784–787.

22. Source obtained from the Internet: Wayne B. Jonas, M.D., "Alternative Medicine: Learning from the Past, Examining the Present, Advancing to the Future," *JAMA*, vol. 280, no. 18 (November 11, 1998): JonasW@od1em.1.od.nih.gov. J. C. Worton, "The history of complementary and alternative medicine," *Essentials of Complementary and Alternative Medicine*, W. B. Jonas and J. H. Levin, eds. (Baltimore, MD: Williams & Wilkins, Inc., In press). T. J. Kaptchuk, "Intentional ignorance: the history of blind assessment and placebo controls in medicine," *Bull Hist Med* 72 (1998): 389–433.

23. CSICOP/News/Scientists and Physicians Gather in Philadelphia for "Science Meets Alternative Medicine."

24. Source obtained from the Internet: Lucette Lagnado, "Oxford to Create Alternative-Medicine Network," *The Wall Street Journal*; www.lightparty.com.

25. K. R. Pelletier, A. Maria, M. Krasner, W. L. Haskell, "Current trends in the integration and reimbursement of complementary and alternative medicine by managed care, insurance carriers, and hospital providers," *Am J Health Promot* 12 (1997): 112–123.

26. Anonymous, "Wasted Health Dollars," *Consumer Reports* (July 1992): 435.

27. Contreras, *Health in the 21st Century*, 209.

28. Charles Inlander, Lowell S. Levin and Ed Weiner, *Medicine on Trial: The appalling story of medical ineptitude and the arrogance that overlooks it* (New York: Pantheon Books, 1988), 113–114.

29. Contreras, *Health in the 21st Century*, 212.

30. Worton, "The history of complementary and alternative medicine." A. Furnham and J. Forey, "The attitudes, behaviors and beliefs of patients of conventional vs. complementary (alternative) medicine," *J Clin Psychol* 50 (1994): 458–469. J. A. Astin, "Why patients use alternative medicine: results of a national study," *JAMA* 279 (1998): 1548–1553.

31. Worton, "The history of complementary and alternative medicine." A. Antonovsky, *Unraveling the Mystery of Health: How People Manage Stress and Stay Well* (San Francisco, CA: Jossey-Bass; 1987).

32. S. Smith, M. Freeland, S. Heffler and D. McKusick, "The Next Ten Years of Health Spending," *Health Aff* 17 (1998): 128–140.

33. Contreras, *Health in the 21st Century,* 227.
34. D. S. Sobel, "Rethinking medicine: improving health outcomes with cost-effective psychosocial interventions," *Psychosom Med* 57 (1995): 234–244. Jonas, "Alternative Medicine: Learning from the Past, Examining the Present, Advancing to the Future."

Chapter 12: Faith for the Coming Cancer Cure

1. Alice Calaprice, ed., *The Quotable Einstein* (Princeton, NJ: Princeton University Press, 1996), 147.
2. Gerald L. Schroeder, *The Science of God* (New York: Broadway Books, Bantam Doubleday Dell Publishing, 1997), 93.
3. Arthur Peacocke, *Paths From Science Towards God* (Oxford, England: Oneworld, 2001), xv.
4. Schroeder, *The Science of God,* 3.
5. Fred Heeren, *Show Me God* (Wheeling, IL: Day Star Publications, 1998), 92.
6. Ibid., 93.
7. Ibid.
8. Peacocke, *Paths From Science Towards God,* 142.

Appendix B: The AIDS Dilemma

1. Adrienne S. Gaines, "A Continent in Crisis," *Charisma* (March 2001): 82.
2. Ibid.
3. Source obtained from the Internet: Jon Jeter, "South Africa AIDS Drug Suit," *Washington Post* (March 6, 2001): www.washingtonpost.com/wpdyn/articles/A26902-2001Mar5.html.
4. Ibid.
5. Ibid.
6. Gaines, "A Continent in Crisis," 82.

Appendix C: Business Interests

1. Werth, *The Billion Dollar Molecule,* 20.
2. Ibid.
3. Contreras, *Health in the 21st Century,* 166.
4. Doug Podolsky and Rita Rubin, "Heal thyself," *U.S. News and World Report* (November 22, 1993): 64–76.

Appendix D: Consequences of the System

1. Beasley, *The Betrayal of Health,* 199.

2. Robert Mendelsohn, *Confessions of a Medical Heretic* (Chicago: Contemporary Books, 1979), 28.
3. Randy Shilts, *And the Band Played On: Politics, people and the AIDS epidemic* (New York: Penguin Books, 1988), 25.
4. Beasley, *The Betrayal of Health*, 200.
5. Werth, *The Billion Dollar Molecule*, 58.
6. Mendelsohn, *Confessions of a Medical Heretic*, 33.
7. Ibid., 34.
8. John Robbins, *Reclaiming Our Health: Exploding the Medical Myth and Embracing the Source of True Healing* (California: Tiburon, 1996), 160.

Appendix E: Modern Research Proves Significance of Diet

1. Gerald T. Keusch, Carla S. Wilson and Samuel E. Waksal, *Nutrition, Host Defenses, and the Lymphoid System; Advances in Host Defense Mechanisms*, vol. 2 (New York: Raven Press, 1983).
2. Robert Good, Gabriel Fernandes and Noorbibi D. Day, *The Influence of Nutrition on Development of Cancer Immunity and Resistance to Mesenchymal Diseases: Molecular Interrelations of Nutrition and Cancer* (New York: Raven Press, 1982).
3. Eduardo N. Siguel, "Cancerostatic Effect of Vegetarian Diets," *Nutrition and Cancer* 4 (1983): 285–289.

Appendix F: Contamination of Water Supplies

1. Contreras, *Health in the 21st Century*, 61–62.
2. Beasley, *The Betrayal of Health*, 100.
3. Contreras, *Health in the 21st Century*, 62.
4. Beasley, *The Betrayal of Health*, 117–118.
5. Ibid., 113.

Appendix G: Nuclear Contamination

1. Ibid., 128.
2. Contreras, *Health in the 21st Century*, 79.
3. Susuki and Knudtson, *Genetica*.
4. Ibid.
5. Ibid.
6. Source obtained from the Internet: raleigh.dis.anl.gov/new/-findingaids/epidemiologic/hanford/intro.html.

Appendix H: Issel's Cancer Treatment

1. Source obtained from the Internet: www.issels.com.

If you enjoyed *The Coming Cancer Cure,* here are some other titles from Siloam Press that can help you to live in health—body, mind and spirit...

A Healthy Heart
Francisco Contreras, M.D.
ISBN: 0-88419-765-4
Retail Price: $19.99

Even if you've never experienced heart problems, you need to read this book. In it noted oncologist Dr. Francisco Contreras shares his medical expertise and wisdom as he explains the causes and treatments for heart disease. You will learn why technology can't always help, and you'll discover powerful keys for reclaiming heart health.

Walking in Divine Health
Don Colbert, M.D.
ISBN: 0-88419-626-7
Price: $10.99

Now you can know what foods have the potential to poison your body and what foods provide the greatest nutritional benefits for good health. Dr. Colbert thoroughly discusses the use of vitamins and minerals, giving many natural sources by which we can maintain our dietary needs for these substances.

Breaking the Grip of Dangerous Emotions
Janet Maccaro, Ph.D., C.N.C.
ISBN: 0-88419-749-2
Retail Price: $19.99

Learn how to stop letting dangerous emotions rob you of your joy as you discover the truth about worry and stress. You can replenish your physical body with a cutting-edge nutritional program that will restore your health. Explore exciting and proven protocols for rebuilding and regenerating your body, mind and spirit.

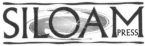
SILOAM PRESS
Living in Health—Body, Mind and Spirit

To pick up a copy of any of these titles, contact your local Christian bookstore or order online at www.charismawarehouse.com.

Your Walk With God Can Be Even Deeper...

With *Charisma* magazine, you'll be informed and inspired by the features and stories about what the Holy Spirit is doing in the lives of believers today.

Each issue:

- Brings you exclusive world-wide reports to rejoice over.
- Keeps you informed on the latest news from a Christian perspective.
- Includes miracle-filled testimonies to build your faith.
- Gives you access to relevant teaching and exhortation from the most respected Christian leaders of our day.

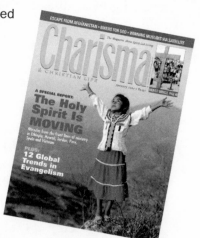

Call 1-800-829-3346 for 3 FREE trial issues

Offer #A2CCHB

If you like what you see, then pay the invoice of $22.97 (**saving over 51% off the cover price**) and receive 9 more issues (12 in all). Otherwise, write "cancel" on the invoice, return it, and owe nothing.

Experience the Power of Spirit-Led Living

Charisma
& CHRISTIAN LIFE

Charisma Offer #A2CCHB
P.O. Box 420234
Palm Coast, Florida 32142-0234
www.charismamag.com

1884A